DIAGNOSTIC TESTS FOR WOMEN

SO-BKP-504

Meet Dr. Readmore. She'll be dispensing additional advice and interesting facts alongside the descriptions of the tests, the procedures involved, and the results of the tests in this section of the book.

INTRODUCTION

You probably have this book in your hands because your doctor has recommended that you have a diagnostic test, and you want to know more about what you will experience. **Many women will have skipped this introduction and opened the page for the test they are going to take.** That's fine. But if you would like to know a little more about medical diagnostic tests for women in general, or about the suggested tests for women at different ages, read on.

Some words of reassurance

The great majority of screening tests recommended for women by doctors are routine preventive measures to be certain that your body is healthy and functioning normally. These tests are important because even most of the serious diseases can be cured or controlled when discovered in early stages. But they are not cause for alarm or anxiety. A few of the routine tests are uncomfortable, embarrassing, or as painful as the sting of a hypodermic needle. Most are minimally invasive and painless. The best news of all is that the vast majority of all preventive tests reveal that the patient is healthy and problem-free.

An overview of medical testing for women

Just a few years ago, two-thirds of all clinical trial participants were men, and it was assumed that research findings would apply equally to women. However, **distinct biological differences have been found in women's and men's organs and organ systems,** including the heart, brain, bones, skin, and saliva, and certain diseases affect one sex but not the other, or affect the two sexes differently.

It was not until 1993 that the National Institutes of Health (NIH) required researchers receiving federal funds to include women in clinical trials. The term gender-specific biology was not coined until 1995. In 1997, the NIH initiated a 15-year, $628 million study to look at women's health issues. Included in the study are trials to prevent heart disease, osteoporosis, breast and colorectal cancer in women. Although the study is still in its earliest stages, there is now a heightened awareness of gender-specific biology within the medical profession as a whole, and among health researchers in particular.

Specifically, doctors have become more vigilant in testing women for cardiovascular disease, lung cancer, breast cancer, cervical cancer, and osteoporosis. Heart attacks are approximately twice as likely to be fatal in women than in men. Although 80% of lung cancer and other pulmonary disease is directly linked to tobacco use, young women continue to smoke at alarming rates. Women are more prone than men to depression, problems with reproductive organs, knee ligament injuries, liver damage from alcohol, and bone loss. Women are eight times as likely to contract HIV from one act of intercourse as men. Grave's Disease, a thyroid hormone disorder, affects seven times as many women as men.

Issues in testing for women

The largest single problem in medical testing is fear —not fear of the generally painless tests themselves, but of the results.
Happily, 61% of all American women have an annual physical exam; 66% a breast exam; and 64% a Pap Test. Approximately 61% of American women 50 years and old have had a mammogram. The motivating factor for most women is the ease of mind provided by good reports or the early detection of problems.

Despite careful laboratory procedures and skilled diagnostic analysts, **test results can be incorrect.** In most cases in which an abnormality is detected, a doctor will order the same test again, or another test for verification. Because of both technical and procedural problems, Pap tests are prone to false positives or negatives, and may be re-tested multiple times in a short period for women with particular symptoms or risk factors.

An additional important issue is the interpretation of test results. If your doctor diagnoses a condition based on tests, you must have a discussion with him or her about the medical evidence he or she has found and feel comfortable asking about the possibility of error. If you are not completely confident in the answers you receive, do not hesitate to seek a second opinion. Particularly in the diagnosis of life-threatening diseases, the majority of doctors will welcome consultation with a colleague.

Finally, it's up to you.

Your best assurance of thorough, competent testing, however, is your own cooperation and communication with doctors and technicians. You should initiate a dialogue about the testing and ask questions about the procedures. **Read the information in this book and be empowered. Take responsibility for your own health.**

These are the
SECTIONS
*in the book.
At the end of
each section
there are
references
for more
information
about specific
tests or
conditions.
Also listed at the
end of each
section are web
sites and
addresses of
organizations
dealing with
health and
diagnostic
testing.*

more

What are the tests, and

6

As medical technology advances, new diagnostic tests become available to consumers, often before they become accepted procedures by the medical profession. Recent developments include the combination of sophisticated computer analysis and various imaging methods to provide fast, noninvasive, three-dimensional views inside all parts of a body—all for a price. For example, a full body scan using electron-beam computed tomography costs approximately $500 to $725. A PET scan which screens your body by function rather than by structure can run as much as $2,000 to $3,000. Low dose CT scans which are often used to study a specific organ, say the lungs, are a bargain at $200 to $300. Critics argue that these tests engender unnecessary expense, cause undue worry to healthy people, and have no measurable benefit for the majority of people tested. Few insurance companies will pay for these scans as preventive tests. However, if you are willing to pay, there is no better way to visualize what is happening inside your body.

What tests should you take

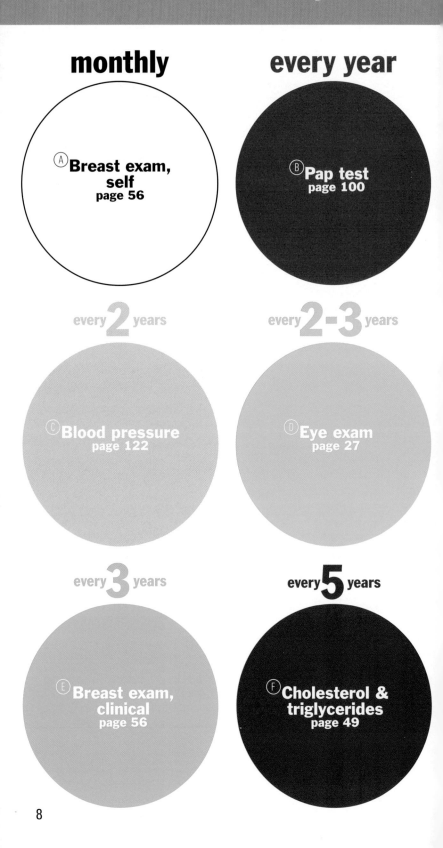

monthly

Ⓐ **Breast exam, self**
page 56

every year

Ⓑ **Pap test**
page 100

every **2** years

Ⓒ **Blood pressure**
page 122

every **2-3** years

Ⓓ **Eye exam**
page 27

every **3** years

Ⓔ **Breast exam, clinical**
page 56

every **5** years

Ⓕ **Cholesterol & triglycerides**
page 49

Where
the test
will be
performed

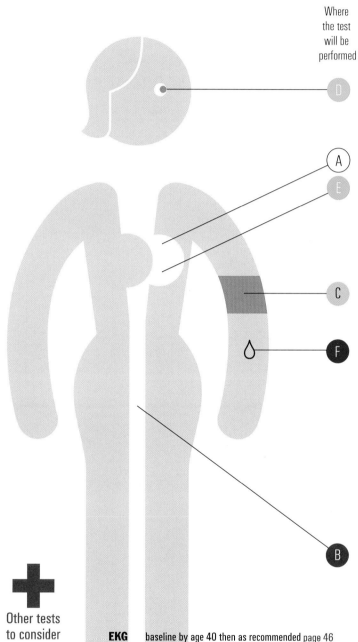

Other tests
to consider

EKG	baseline by age 40 then as recommended page 46	
Urinalysis	as directed by your doctor page 75	
Bone Densitometry	baseline at menopause, then as recommended page 112	
Complete blood count	as directed by your doctor page 123	
Skin exam	20-39 every **3** years, 40+ every **year**	
exually transmitted disease screen	as directed by your doctor	

9

monthly

Breast exam,
self
page 56

every year

B Mammogram
page 54

C Breast exam, clinical
page 56

D Pap test
page 100

every 2 years

E Eye exam
page 27

F Blood pressure
page 122

every 3 years

starting
at age 45

G Glucose
(blood sugar)
page 83

every 5 years

H Cholesterol &
triglycerides
page 49

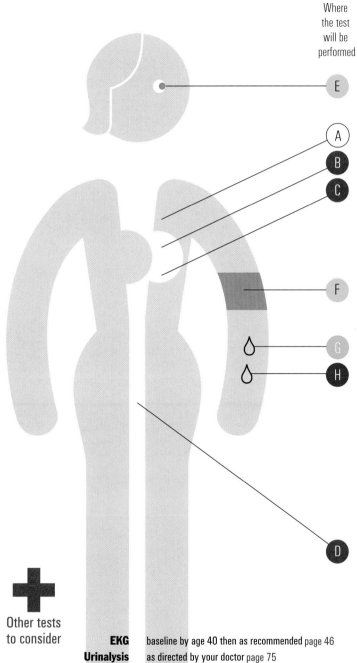

Where the test will be performed

E

A

B

C

F

G

H

D

Other tests to consider

EKG	baseline by age 40 then as recommended	page 46
Urinalysis	as directed by your doctor	page 75
Bone Densitometry	baseline at menopause, then as recommended	page 112
Complete blood count	as directed by your doctor	page 123
Skin exam	every **year**	
Sexually transmitted disease screen	as directed by your doctor	

What tests should you take

monthly

(A) **Breast exam, self**
page 56

every year

(B) **Mammogram**
page 54

(C) **Breast exam, clinical**
page 56

(D) **Pap test**
page 100

(E) **Fecal occult blood**
page 94

every 2 years

(F) **Eye exam**
page 27

(G) **Blood pressure**
page 122

every 3 years

(H) **Glucose**
(blood sugar)
page 83

every 3-5 years

(J) **Colon exam**
pages 94–95

**Sigmoidoscopy,
Colonoscopy
or Colon X-ray**
(Colonoscopy is most
comprehensive but may not be
covered by insurance.)

every 5 years

(K) **Cholesterol &
triglycerides**
page 49

(L) **Digital rectal exam**
page 97

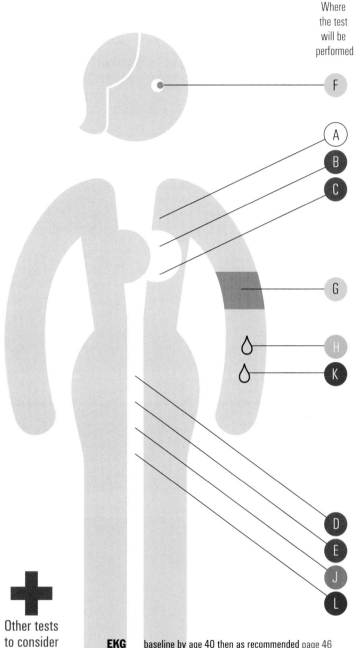

Where the test will be performed

F

A

B

C

G

H

K

D

E

J

L

Other tests to consider

EKG	baseline by age 40 then as recommended page 46	
Urinalysis	as directed by your doctor page 75	
Bone Densitometry	baseline at menopause, then as recommended page 112	
Complete blood count	as directed by your doctor page 123	
Skin exam	every year	
Sexually transmitted disease screen	as directed by your doctor	

13

What tests should you take

monthly

(A) **Breast exam,
self**
page 56

every year

(B) **Eye exam**
page 27

(C) **Mammogram**
page 54

(D) **Breast exam, clinical**
page 56

(E) **Pap test**
page 100

(F) **Fecal occult blood**
page 94

every 2 years

(G) **Blood pressure**
page 122

every 3 years

(H) **Glucose**
(blood sugar)
page 83

every 3-5 years

(J) **Colon exam**
pages 94–95

Sigmoidoscopy,
Colonoscopy
or Colon X-ray

(Colonoscopy is most
comprehensive but may not be
covered by insurance.)

every 5 years

(K) **Cholesterol &
triglycerides**
page 49

(L) **Digital rectal exam**
page 97

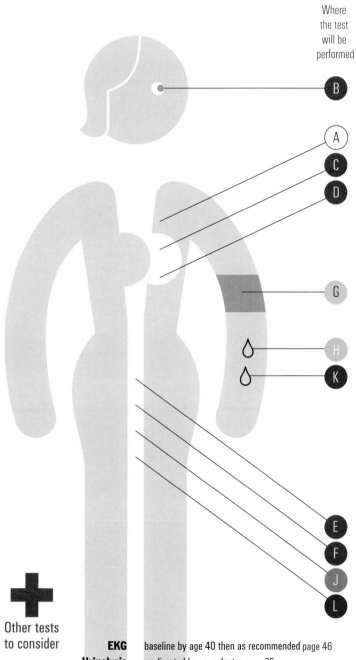

Where
the test
will be
performed

B

A

C

D

G

H

K

E

F

J

L

Other tests
to consider

EKG	baseline by age 40 then as recommended page 46
Urinalysis	as directed by your doctor page 75
Bone Densitometry	baseline at menopause, then as recommended page 112
Complete blood count	as directed by your doctor page 123
Skin exam	every **year**
exually transmitted disease screen	as directed by your doctor

15

What tests should you take

monthly

(A) **Breast exam, self**
page 56

every year

(B) **Eye exam**
page 27

(C) **Mammogram**
page 54

(D) **Breast exam, clinical**
page 56

(E) **Pap test**
page 100

(F) **Fecal occult blood**
page 94

every 2 years

(G) **Blood pressure**
page 122

every 3 years

(H) **Glucose**
(blood sugar)
page 83

every 3-5 years

(J) **Colon exam**
pages 94–95

**Sigmoidoscopy,
Colonoscopy
or Colon X-ray**

(Colonoscopy is most
comprehensive but may not be
covered by insurance.)

every 5 years

(K) **Cholesterol &
triglycerides**
page 49

(L) **Digital rectal exam**
page 97

Where
the test
will be
performed

B

A

C

D

G

H

K

E

F

J

L

Other tests
to consider

EKG	baseline by age 40 then as recommended page 46
Urinalysis	as directed by your doctor page 75
Bone Densitometry	baseline at menopause, then as recommended page 112
Complete blood count	as directed by your doctor page 123
Skin exam	every **year**
exually transmitted disease screen	as directed by your doctor

17

At birth, the human brain weighs about three-quarters of a pound, and certain areas of the newborn forebrain show no electrical activity at all until the age of seven or eight months. The average **adult** brain weighs approximately three pounds. There is no correlation between normal variations in human brain size and intelligence.

The brain is the major organ of the nervous system, and the primary computer of the human body. It is composed of more than one hundred billion nerve cells, each of which is connected to thousands of others, which make it far more complex than any mere computer— and more sensitive.

Brain disorders are treated by a neurologist, who specializes in problems of the nervous system. These problems may have either physical or behavioral manifestations. Many brain-related disorders such as mental retardation, are evident at birth, though some may develop during life. Other disorders include stroke, brain tumor, blood vessel abnormalities (aneurysms), epilepsy/seizures, migraines headaches, and other neurological diseases.

Cancers of the brain are among the most common brain diseases. They affect not only the brain itself, but also the part of the body regulated by the region of the brain impaired by the tumor. This unique aspect of the brain—its function as the control center of the systems of the body—makes treatment a sensitive issue.

From middle age onward, the most important threat to the brain is impaired blood supply to one or more brain regions, which causes the death of irreplaceable brain cells. If an artery within the brain becomes blocked or ruptures, causing hemorrhage, the result is called a *stroke*. Risk factors for stroke include age, high blood

pressure, arteriosclerosis (plaque buildup in arteries), diabetes, and smoking. Stroke kills approximately 144,000 people in the United States annually, 60% of whom are women.

Alzheimer's disease (AD) is the most common cause of dementia in older people. The disease usually begins after age 65, and the risk of AD goes up with age. It affects about 3 percent of men and women aged 65 to 74, and nearly half of those over age 85 may have the disease. Nevertheless, **Alzheimer's is not a normal characteristic of old age.**

Some disorders of the brain affect women more than men. Migraine headaches are a severe, throbbing pain over one or both temples, or behind one eye or ear, and are often accompanied by nausea and vomiting. 20 million women in the U.S. suffer from headaches, nine million of whom suffer debiliting migraines.

Over a quarter of women are affected by migraines during their life.

The prevalence of migraine is two to three times higher in women than in men, probably due to hormonal differences. Women also report higher levels of pain, longer duration of headaches, and more associated symptoms, such as nausea and vomiting. Harvard medical School researchers found in one study that subjects who reported migraines were 80% more likely to have a stroke than those who did not.

There is a long recognized association between estrogen and migraine. Over half of women with migraine report an association between their headaches and their menstrual cycle. The frequency and severity of migraine is increased commonly with the use of oral contraceptives and during menopause.

6 QUESTIONS TO ASK YOUR DOCTOR

? If I think I have a problem with my brain, what should I do right away?

? What is the best test to diagnose my particular symptoms?

? Are there any conditions (such as pregnancy) that would make a particular test a bad idea?

? Are there any restrictions on my diet or activities before the test?

? Does the clinic or hospital require a patient consent form in order to take this test?

? How will I feel after the test?

THE TESTS

CHEMICAL MESSAGE CENTERS

Major glands in the body's endocrine (hormone-producing) system

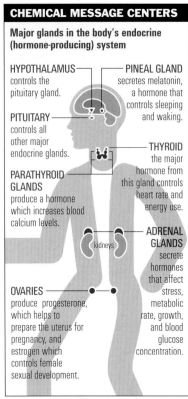

HYPOTHALAMUS controls the pituitary gland.

PINEAL GLAND secretes melatonin, a hormone that controls sleeping and waking.

PITUITARY controls all other major endocrine glands.

THYROID the major hormone from this gland controls heart rate and energy use.

PARATHYROID GLANDS produce a hormone which increases blood calcium levels.

kidneys

ADRENAL GLANDS secrete hormones that affect stress, metabolic rate, growth, and blood glucose concentration.

OVARIES produce progesterone, which helps to prepare the uterus for pregnancy, and estrogen which controls female sexual development.

Hormone Testing

The presence of hormones in the blood and urine is regulated in part by the brain and its subsidiary organs. Too much or too little of various hormones can be signs of brain malfunction. Hormones in the blood may be functionally important, and hormones in the urine may signify disease.

Procedure

Blood and urine—collected in the usual manner—can both be tested for hormones moving through the body. Blood or urine samples may require fasting or may need to be taken early in the morning, depending on the hormone. In certain cases, 24 hour urine testing may be required.

Results

High or low levels of cortisol in the blood indicate malfunction of the pituitary or adrenal glands. Often this suggests a tumor in one of these glands. Testosterone, while it is associated

with males, is produced in some quantities by both sexes, so each has a normal range. Anything outside of this range indicates malfunction of the pituitary gland. Tumors can cause this malfunction, as can a malfunctioning thyroid (*See* **THROAT** *pages 41-42*). Pituitary hormones regulate much of the body, particularly the reproductive functions. These include the hormones which trigger menstruation such as the luteinizing hormone (LH) and follicle stimulating hormone (FSH). Malfunctions in these organs lead to testing these hormones in the blood. Again, tumors or a malfunctioning thyroid may be the cause.

Spinal Tap or Lumbar Puncture

In this test, fluid which flows around the brain and spine is withdrawn for analysis.

Procedure

An area in the lower back or back of the neck is anesthetized and sterilized. A needle in then inserted into the lower back between two vertebrae to withdraw the fluid that bathes the brain and spinal cord. This fluid flows up and down the spinal column and around the brain, as well. Proper insertion may require several tries and can be painful.

Results

The cerebrospinal fluid is a leading indicator of problems in the brain and spine. It is usually clear, and the presence of almost any type of cells in the fluid can indicate infection or leakage from the brain. The fluid's pressure may be taken as well.

Cerebrospinal fluid may be tested for:

Alzheimer's Disease

The presence of Amyloid Beta Protein can be an indication of Alzheimer's and other dementias.

WHAT ALZHEIMER'S LOOKS LIKE
Sections through two brains

NORMAL

ALZHEIMER'S
showing
cell death

Many tests and a large overview are often needed to diagnose Alzheimer's. A.D. is a clinical diagnosis, not a laboratory test diagnosis.

An estimated 4 million people in the U.S. suffer from Alzheimer's Disease. Alzheimer's begins with forgetfulness and the inability to do simple tasks, such as math problems. These difficulties build with time, and the ability to think clearly diminishes as well. Speaking, understanding, reading, writing, and caring for oneself all fade slowly as well.

Bleeding
Detection of red blood cells may indicate bleeding from an aneurysm.

Meningitis
The fluid may be examined under a microscope or cultured to test for meningitis, an infection of the meniges (the membranes that cover the brain and spinal cord.)

Multiple Sclerosis
If certain proteins are found, MS may be diagnosed.

Computerized Axial Tomography (CAT or CT Scan)
This type of scan can be useful anywhere on the body, but particularly on the brain. It provides sharp, two and three dimensional images of the brain and can be used to localize tumors, clots or other brain abnormalities.

Procedure
In the case of the brain CAT scan, the patient lies on a table which moves into the scanner. The patient must lie motionless while the scanner takes pictures, for up to an hour. Sometimes an iodine contrast dye is injected, which can help obtain clearer pictures. Although rare in the newer, fast scanners, and scanners that are "open" on the sides, some patients experience claustrophobia and may require a sedative.

Results
Symptoms such as headaches, dizziness, seizures, extremity weakness or numbness usually lead to this test. Possible causes of these problems that this test can detect are brain tumors, evidence of a stroke, or treatable causes of dementia.

CAT SCAN MACHINE

The patient lies on a table which is moved slowly into the scanner gantry. This houses a rotating x-ray tube and receptors and can make a series of 30 images in a few seconds.

Doppler Ultrasound
This type of ultrasound is particularly capable of detecting motion, such as blood flow in veins and arteries. It may show arterial narrowing or blockages.

Procedure
As with all ultrasounds, a hand-held probe is passed over the area of inter-

est and the sound waves are converted to a picture. In this case, large vessel blood flow to the brain can be observed.

Results

The technician or doctor can see and report immediately any abnormalities that are observed. Clots, arterial plaques or obstructions that cause strokes can be detected, along with blood flow patterns in the brain which can show evidence of dead tissue in parts of the brain.

Electroencephalography (EEG, Brain Wave Test)

This painless test measures the electrical impulses produced by the brain, which usually appear in a normal pattern. In order to measure electrical activity in the brain, electrodes wired to a machine are applied to the scalp, and readings are taken. Abnormal brain wave patterns can assist the doctor in diagnosing brain tumors, stroke, blood clots, epilepsy and seizures.

Procedure

The patient lies down, and up to 30 electrodes are adhered to the scalp with conductive gel. These are attached to a machine which graphs brain activity over time. The patient lies still, may be shown bright lights, put to sleep with a sedative, or asked to breathe heavily as the machine takes readings. This test lasts up to an hour, at which time the electrodes are removed. The electricity flows from the brain to the machine; there is no risk that it may be reversed.

Results

Abnormal patterns in the EEG waves can indicate brain tumors in a specific area, evidence of a stroke, blood clot or epilepsy, but the most common use is to detect seizures or brain malfunction. The test is also used to establish whether a person is brain-dead.

A variation of this test, called an Evoked Potential Study, provides external stimulus to the brain during

EEG: BRAIN WAVE TESTING

ELECTRODES
(You don't have to shave before they are attached.)

the EEG. The brain is tested to see how quickly it responds. Any significant time lapse can indicate brain damage or damage to the optic nerve or nerves to the ears.

Electromyography

This test examines the function of nerves in the body. In particular, it investigates the electrical pathways between the brain and the muscles it controls.

Procedure

The patient must lie on a table, and electrodes are adhered with gel to the nerve pathway or muscles to be tested. These are attached to a meter which measures electrical current. As the patient tenses and relaxes certain muscles, the electrical output is measured. Under any circumstances, this test is uncomfortable. However, current may be passed between the electrodes as well to stimulate the muscles, which briefly may produce a burning sensation.

Results

The results of this test appear in three ways: on a graph similar to an EEG graph, on a monitor, and as popping noises over a loudspeaker as the nerves fire. The doctor can interpret this collection of data, detecting nerve and brain disease which damages muscle function. Diseases such as multiple sclerosis, myopathy, diabetes, polio, and ALS (Lou Gehrig's Disease) may be diagnosed. This test is usually ordered with signs of muscle weakness or pain.

Magnetic Resonance Imaging (MRI)

This test can be performed on most parts of the body and provides excellent magnetic images, but is particularly useful for the brain. When the results are viewed, tumors, aneurysms, multiple sclerosis and infection are clearly visible.

Procedure

As with all MRIs, the patient lies on the MRI table, which slides into the machine. The patient lies still as the imager thumps and moves around for 30 to 90 minutes. In some cases, just before the test begins, a safe contrast dye may be injected in a vein to provide greater clarity. Although perfect-

ly safe, the MRI imager is disconcertingly more noisy than a CAT scan, and some patients may feel claustrophobic and require a sedative or an "open" scanner.

Results

The images produced are examined by a doctor, who can see the entire area examined. Tumors, aneurysms, blood clots, blood flow, and hemorrhages will be clear to a trained specialist.

MAGNETIC RESONANCE IMAGING

The table slides into the machine.

Octreotide Scan

This nuclear test is used to investigate the status of known tumors, primarily brain tumors.

Procedure

A radioactive substance (sometimes called a radionuclide) is injected into a vein, from which it spreads through the body. This substance is absorbed in greater concentrations by different types of tissue, so that the tissues can be distinguished by a sensitive type of machine that reads levels of radiation, called a gamma camera. This gamma camera (which translates the x-ray-like gamma rays into images) can take pictures of the entire body and show different tissues in clear contrast. Unlike the dyes that are used in cardiac catheterization or coronary angiography, radionuclides carry vir-

CHOICES AMONG BRAIN TESTS: CAT VS. MRI VS. PET

The CAT scan, although it involves slightly more radiation than a normal X-ray, can produce clear images of the brain in less than half an hour. The MRI is exceptionally safe. It involves no radiation and usually no contrast dyes. It can produce images of the brain, blood vessels and some detail of the skull. However, it is an especially expensive test. PET scans produce unusually precise images of brain activity based on metabolic activity. This sophisticated technique allows doctors to "see" brain activity in real time as thoughts are developing. Unfortunately, the cost of PET scans is prohibitive, because the radioisotopes must be produced in a cyclotron.

more tests ▸

tually no risk of toxicity or allergic reaction.

Results

The pictures track the radioactive substance through the body. If the radionuclide has attached to tumors, these should be apparent in the pictures. Tumors can be found and their progress monitored with this test.

Positron Emission Tomography Scan (PET)

This imaging test combines techniques from two common forms of tests: the nuclear scan and biochemical assessment.

Procedure

This test begins with the inhalation or injection of a radioactive element through an IV. Often, a second IV line is required to obtain serial blood samples periodically during the test. The radioactive element, as it decays in the body, emits nuclear energy when metabolized. The patient lies on a table which slides, like a CAT scan, into a large scanning device. The energy can then be measured by scanners. The speed at which the nuclear energy is released allows doctors to observe the metabolism of the patient. The energy emitted can be traced to specific organs, and images can be made based on the speed and location of this energy. This test may sound frightening, but it is safe, nontoxic, and subject to the mild discomfort or claustrophobia of any scan test. Also, recent use of caffeine, alcohol, or tobacco—or brain-influencing drugs such as tranquilizers—may affect test results.

Results

PET traces the distribution pattern of the radioactive substances injected, and translates this information into color pictures. Like the CAT or MRI scans, the PET is used to search for unusual masses in the body. It detects

them by the speed at which they attract and metabolize the nuclear element in the body. Tumors, as well as evidence of heart attacks and strokes, can be seen. Single Photon Emission Computed Tomography (SPECT) is a similar type of test, which uses slightly different technology. SPECT scanning recognizes abnormal cells by their abnormal metabolism, not by their abnormal appearance.

LEFT BRAIN, RIGHT BRAIN

The brain is divided into left and right hemispheres that specialize in different forms of activity. The hemispheres are connected by the **corpus callosum**, a bridge of a hundred million nerve fibers **(shown in red)**. Differences in hemispheric specialization develop in individuals between birth and age 12.

top view

front view, sliced through

SYMPTOMS OF STROKE

The most common stroke symptoms, too often ignored, include

- dizziness
- sudden loss of consciousness
- confusion
- double vision or sudden deterioration in vision
- slurring of speech
- partial paralysis or numbness
- pregnant women also may experience severe headaches, nausea, or seizures.

TOP WAYS TO AVOID A STROKE

Control your **blood pressure** with appropriate medication.

Don't smoke

Take one **aspirin** per day (in consultation with your doctor).

Treat **heart rhythm** problems with vigilance.

Practice a regular routine of proper diet and **exercise**.

Treatment within three hours of a stroke can make the difference between permanent disability or death and normal function. The more quickly you react to stroke symptoms in yourself or others, the more likely you may be able to minimize permanent damage.

For further information

Alzheimer's Association
Suite 1000
919 North Michigan Ave.
Chicago, IL 60611-1676
800-272-3900
www.alz.org

National Headache Foundation
Dept. PF
5252 N. Western Ave.
Chicago, IL 60625
778-878-7715

American Council for Headache
Education
800-255-ACHE
www.cs.uu.ne/wais/html/na-bng/
alt.support.headaches.migraine

National Stroke Association
96 Inverness Drive East
Suite I
Englewood, CO 80112-5112
1-800-STROKES (1-800-787-6537)
www.stroke.org

National Institute of Neurological
Disorders and Stroke
Information Office
P.O. Box 5801
Bethesda, MD 20824
1-800-352-9424

Neurosciences on the Internet
www.neuroguide.com

The Parkinson's Web
www.pdweb.mgh.harvard.edu

Dana BrainWeb
www.dana.org/brainweb

EYES

The normal human eye blinks about 25 times each minute. Eyestrain from working on the computer or reading too long may be the result of insufficient blinking.

The poet who said that "the eyes are the windows of the soul" was only half right. They are windows into the workings of the body, too.

All ophthalmologists and optometrists study ways in which the eyes reflect the health of the entire system. An examination of the arteries and veins visible in the back of the eye can reveal signs of high blood pressure, arteriosclerosis, brain disease, diabetes, and other problems throughout the body. **Diabetes is often linked to vision problems at all ages,** and is the leading cause of blindness in adults between the ages of 20 and 74. It accounts for over 8,000 new cases of blindness each year. Other vision problems may be evident from birth. Babies born prematurely are often vision-impaired, and some full term babies need glasses in infancy. The availability of laser surgery provides the opportunity for permanent vision correction

6 TOP QUESTIONS TO ASK YOUR EYE CARE PROFESSIONAL ABOUT YOUR GENERAL HEALTH

- Do the arteries look healthy and normal?
- Is there any suggestion of high blood pressure?
- Is there any evidence of developing diabetes?
- Are my eyes in good health for my age?
- Can you observe normal optic reflexes?
- Are any blood clots visible?

and is becoming increasingly common. These
vision surgeries, used to treat nearsightedness,
farsightedness and astigmatism, are expensive
but usually accurate one-time fixes—however,
laser surgery can have complications and requires careful consultation
with your eye care professional before deciding to proceed.

Light travels from the optic nerve to the back of the brain at 300 miles per hour.

Most tests for the eyes are simple, painless, and noninvasive.

A few of the more sophisticated
tests for macular degeneration or optic nerve damage may require
hospital-based x-ray or scanning technology, but most eye diagnostics
are conducted by eye care professionals during regular office visits.

During a routine checkup, the patient goes to a private room, and
drops are often put into the patient's eyes. These drops dilate the
pupils, opening them wider so that the inner workings of the eye
and the back, called the retina, are easier to observe. As a result,
these drops may blur vision and make the eye sensitive to light.
Driving, reading and any activity in bright sunlight should be avoided
for several hours after the drops are administered. Patients may
want to call ahead to ask if someone else
should drive home. Different drops are also
used to numb the eyes, so that surface tests
can be performed without discomfort;
these do not cause distortion of vision.

THE TESTS

Results

Visual acuity is expressed as a fraction, the top portion of which is always 20, indicating the 20-foot distance from the patient to the Snellen chart. The bottom portion of the fraction compares the patient's eyesight against the norm. Someone with 20/60 vision sees at 20 feet what those with perfect vision can see at 60 feet, and cannot discern the smaller letters on the chart that are clear to someone with 20/20 vision. This simple test is used (often in conjunction with phorometry—see below) to determine accuracy of vision. If reading the chart proves very difficult, it might indicate a more serious problem, such as glaucoma or cataracts.

Visual Acuity

This common test measures how well the eye can see. The Snellen Eye Chart, first used in 1862, still hangs on most physicians' walls, with its large E on top. This test is performed at nearly every general physical, as well as during every visit to an eye care professional.

Procedure

The chart, with its rows of rapidly shrinking letters, is set 20 feet from the patient, who must then read down the chart until the letters are no longer clear. The test is done one eye at a time, and first done without glasses, then with them, if the patient wears them. A chart with other symbols may be used for preschoolers and patients who are not familiar with the Western alphabet.

In addition to distance vision, a Jaeger card is used to test near vision. This card works just like its larger cousin, with rows of letters which decrease in size. The card is placed at a set distance from the patient, who then reads until the letters are no longer clear. The Jaeger card can be used to determine a prescription for reading glasses or bifocals.

Some pet owners will believe anything!

Phorometry

A phoropter is an instrument with many different lenses that test the eyes' ability to focus. Phorometry involves looking at the Snellen Chart (*see above*) through these goggles, which place adjustable lenses in front of the eye.

Procedure

The phoropter is lowered over the face and different lenses are placed between the eye and the chart. The patient is asked to judge which lens makes the letters appear clearer, and the lenses are increasingly fine-tuned as the test goes on. The patient is asked to judge the clarity of vision in each eye for distance and close-up vision.

GETTING THE RIGHT LENSES

The phoropter

Results

The goal of this test is to determine the strength of glasses or contact lenses to be prescribed.

Visual Field Test (Perimetry)

This test measures the sensitivity of your retina to light across different areas of the visual field.

Procedure

The patient rests his head in a chin rest, facing a bowl shaped instrument. A series of lights go on and off and the patient is asked to respond to what is seen.

Results

The absence or reduction of sensitivity in one or more areas may indicate one or more disorders, including glaucoma.

Color Defectiveness Determination

True color blindness, in which everything appears black and white, is relatively rare. Color defectiveness or color deficiency is far more common. This test measures the ability to discern differences among various colors.

Procedure

The test involves looking at a series of slides which have color patterns on them. The patient will be asked to identify what is on the slide.

Results

Within the color patterns are numbers and letters which are obvious to normal eyes, but not to those that are color defective. Several types of color defectiveness exist which make two different colors appear the same. For example, red-green color-blind people cannot distinguish these two colors.

COLOR BLINDNESS

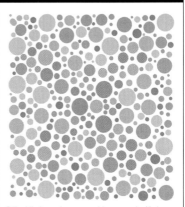

Color blind people are not able to see the X above.

About ten times more men than women are color blind. The most common color deficiency is red/green. Inability to detect the color blue is very rare.

Muscle Integrity Evaluation

This test evaluates the health and function of the muscles which control eye movement.

Procedure

The doctor or technician directs the patient to perform simple motions with the eye—back and forth, up and down. These eye movements are observed by the doctor.

Results

If there is any problem moving the eye, or a discrepancy between the response of one eye and the response

more tests

of the other, it could indicate muscle or nerve damage or deterioration.

The definition of legal blindness in the US is determined in two ways. First, if no better than 20/200 corrected vision can be attained in a person's better eye, he or she is considered legally blind. Second, if a person's tunnel vision is so far advanced that the visual field is restricted to 20 degrees or less, they also are legally blind.

Glaucoma is the second leading cause of irreversible blindness in the US, and the leading cause among African-Americans. The incidence of glaucoma is four to six times higher in blacks than in whites, and it becomes more prevalent with age. Among whites, glaucoma is present in 0.5-1.5% of persons under age 65 and 2-4% of those over 75. Among blacks, 1.2% of those between the ages of 40 and 49 and 11.3% of those over 80 have glaucoma. Prevalence of glaucoma is increased in patients with diabetes mellitus, myopia, and a family history of glaucoma. Of the various forms of glaucoma, primary open-angle glaucoma (POAG) is the most common in the US (80-90% of cases), and is estimated to be responsible for impaired vision in 1.6 million Americans and blindness in 150,000.

Dry Eye Test (Schirmer Tear Test)

This test assesses the functioning of the lacrimal glands in the eye, and measures the quantity of tearing.

Procedure

After the patient is seated comfortably in an examining chair, she is asked to look up and a sterile strip of filter paper is gently inserted under each of the lower eyelids. After a period of time, usually five minutes, the strips are removed from the patient's eyes and the length of the moistened area on the filter paper is measured in millimeters.

Results

A Schirmer test strip should show at least 15 mm of moisture after five min-

utes. Because tear production decreases with age, 10 mm would still be within the normal range for patients over the age of forty. The problem of "dry eyes" is normally associated with aging, although rarely may result from systemic diseases. Up to 15% of the patients taking the Schirmer test have false-positive or false-negative results. Because the test is quick and simple, it is usually repeated to compare results in question.

CHANGING SHAPE

The **pupil**... ...becomes smaller when a bright light is shined into it.

Pupillary Reflex Response

This test measures how fast the pupil closes when confronted by a bright light.

Procedure

Whenever the eye is exposed to bright light, the pupil is supposed to become smaller. A bright light, shined by the doctor or technician into the eye, should trigger this response.

Results

The closure of the pupil in the presence of bright light is a reflex. When light shines into the eye, any abnormality in the response can be an indication of nerve damage, damage to the cornea, or damage to the iris, which controls the pupil.

Keratoconus, a progressive thinning of the cornea, affects one in every 2,000 Americans, and is most prevalent in teenagers and adults in their 20s. It can be detected during routine eye exams and treated with contact lenses in 90% of the cases. Advanced cases may require corneal transplants.

Floaters, which appear to the patient as spots that "float" across the field of vision, can also be a sign of deterioration of the retina, although more often they are normal visual defects that inhibit vision only slightly. New floaters may be associated with a retinal tear or detachment.

Slit Lamp Exam (Biomicroscopy)

The slit lamp is a device which examines the front of the eye. A doctor can see the surface, cornea, and lens up close in order to determine that they are in healthy condition.

Procedure

The eyes are sometimes dilated with drops, and the patient is instructed to sit forward and rest the chin on the slit lamp apparatus. The doctor then moves the lamp around to look into the eye while the patient looks straight ahead. One variation of this test involves introducing fluorescein dye into the eye, either by drops or on a paper strip which is touched to the eye. This dye spreads across the surface of the eye, and stains any cuts, tears, or foreign bodies, making them easy to observe.

Results

The eye should appear normal and healthy. The doctor can see scratches on the surface of the eye, as well as damage to the eyelids, cornea, or lens of the eye. The doctor can also detect infections, inflammations and the presence of foreign objects lodged in the eyeball.

Intraocular Pressure Determination (Tonometry)

This test measures the internal pressure of the eye, and should be performed with each eye examination.

Procedure

After anesthetic drops are put in the eye, the front of the eyeball is touched gently with a pen-like tube, the tip of which measures pressure. This is slightly unnerving but not uncomfortable or painful. A variation on this procedure is the "air puff" tonometry, which requires no direct contact, but can also accurately measure pressure.

Results

High pressure can be an indicator of something wrong within the eye, although not all abnormal pressure indicates glaucoma. Many patients with high pressure (perhaps more than 70%) will never develop vision problems due to glaucoma. However, this test is extremely important as a preventive measure, and early detection can save loss of vision.

More and more, evidence says that tonometry is not as closely related to glaucoma as once thought. High-risk patients may want to seek the newer technology of the Hillelberg Retinal Tomograph.

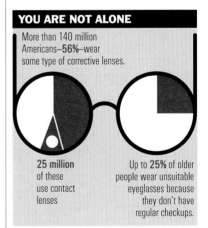

YOU ARE NOT ALONE

More than 140 million Americans—**56%**—wear some type of corrective lenses.

25 million of these use contact lenses

Up to **25%** of older people wear unsuitable eyeglasses because they don't have regular checkups.

Retinal Examination (Direct Ophthalmoscopy or Fundoscopy)

This test is a way for the doctor to examine the inside and rear of the eye. The retina is the only place in the body where blood flow can be noninvasively observed.

more tests ▶

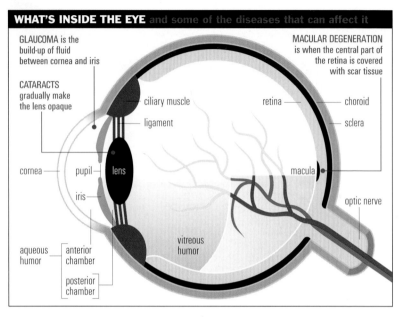

WHAT'S INSIDE THE EYE and some of the diseases that can affect it

GLAUCOMA is the build-up of fluid between cornea and iris

CATARACTS gradually make the lens opaque

MACULAR DEGENERATION is when the central part of the retina is covered with scar tissue

ciliary muscle

ligament

retina — choroid

— sclera

cornea — pupil — lens

iris

macula

optic nerve

aqueous humor | anterior chamber

posterior chamber

vitreous humor

Procedure

Using a small instrument with a small beam light source and magnifying lens (the ophthalmoscope), the doctor peers into the eyes and asks the patient to fix on a point, while the doctor moves the light source for examination. The bright light, especially if the eyes have been dilated, can be uncomfortable to look at.

Results

This test allows the doctor to get an idea of the general health of the body, and may reveal whether a patient has high blood pressure or diabetes. The doctor also can see the retina at the back of the eye and determine whether there is any damage to it. "Floaters" become visible, as does any retinal detachment or the beginning signs of macular degeneration. Although rare, blood clots from a stroke, tumors, or fluid attributed to meningitis infections may be visible as well.

Another version of this test, called Binocular Indirect Ophthalmoscopy, uses brighter light and dilation drops. The doctor uses a lamp which can be attached to the head, or another light source and hand-held magnifying lenses through which light can be shone. By focusing and directing brighter light, more of the eye can be seen, and in greater detail.

Orbital Computerized Tomography Scan

This specialized form of CAT scan (the orbit is a medical term for the eye socket area) may be required for a clearer view of eye anatomy, to determine the cause of abnormal protrusions of the eyeball, or to diagnose brain-related disorders or circulatory disorders. Though standard x-rays of the orbit are often used for similar purposes, the CAT scan gives a more three-dimensional view of the eye and its surrounding structures.

Procedure

As with other CAT scans, the goal is to obtain extremely detailed x-rays. All hair clips, jewelry or other objects are removed. The patient lies flat on a table, and the head is placed in a stabilized, cushioned area which slides into the scanner, a large-doughnut shaped instrument. To ensure clear images, the patient must lie completely still. The scanner moves around the head, clicking and taking pictures which can then be interpreted by a computer and converted into images. Although the test takes half an hour, the patient may become uncomfortable lying stationary on a hard table for this length of time. Often, after the initial scan is completed, a dye is injected into the arm and the scan is repeated (*see also Fluorescein Angiography*).

Results
The scan is looking for brain-related disorders, such as blood clots, nerve damage or tumors, which can manifest themselves in vision problems. This scan may also help doctors to assess eye damage caused by thyroid disease or bony orbit fractures in trauma injuries. If abnormalities such as bumps develop within the eye, the scan can help identify their cause. These may be foreign objects, infections, blood clots or tumors.

Sight deteriorates naturally with time and degenerative disorders become more prevalent with age. The three most common vision problems affecting people over 50 are presbyopia (a natural aspect of aging that blurs the near vision, correctable with reading glasses), glaucoma (a build-up of pressure in the eye that, untreated, can result in blindness), and cataracts (protein build-up causing a clouding of the lenses that surgeons repair by replacing the lens). Periodic check-ups will routinely include tests for these diseases. Their causes are largely unknown, although genetics and overall health contribute to most.

Eye Ultrasonography
The ultrasound can differentiate among tissues of different densities and is thus useful for close observation of the eye, and to test for abnormalities.

Procedure
The patient is seated in a large chair,

and anesthetic drops are placed in each eye. After the room is darkened, an ultrasound transducer, a pen-like device, is touched to the eyeball in several places. Sound waves transported through the eye and back to the device are recorded as images on a screen. This may be slightly uncomfortable, but the time to "sound" both eyes is less than ten minutes.

How to give your eyes a quick rest in the midst of prolonged reading or computer work: Look out a window and/or focus on objects at a distance. Tilt your head back, chin to the ceiling, and roll your head from side-to-side gently with your eyes open. Raise your eyebrows, keep your head still, and look up.

Results
This test can distinguish tumors and other abnormalities from normal tissue in the eye. Ultrasound can also locate and identify any suspected foreign object which might be lodged in the eye

Fluorescein Angiography
This photo process identifies many problems, including retinal infections or other infections deep in the eye. Damage to the blood flow to and within the eye as well as macular degeneration are also detectable using this test. (see angiography in the terms section)

Procedure
Although this test is one of the most serious eye diagnostics, it can cause only slight discomfort. After the eyes have been dilated, fluorescein dye is injected into an arm vein, causing the vessels of the retina to turn bright orange almost immediately. The injection is moderately painful, like a pin prick, and the dye can sting or cause the patient to feel faint. Allergic reactions are possible as well,

more tests ▶

so the patient must disclose all allergies to the doctor. With the patient's chin resting against the camera, bright flash pictures are taken of the eye every few seconds, for about a minute. Because the eyes have been dilated, this brightness will probably be uncomfortable. Afterwards the patient's urine will be colored orange for several days as the dye passes out of the body.

THE AMSLER GRID

As seen by someone with normal vision

As seen by someone with macular degeneration

Macular Degeneration is a disease which has received growing interest from the medical profession in the past few years. The macula, an area in the middle of the retina, starts to lose its light sensitivity, causing the vision to blur. Sometimes this is due to blood vessels growing into the area, which can be treated with laser surgery. Aside from this procedure which may slow its spread, however, there is no cure. It typically occurs in both eyes, but symptoms usually appear in one eye first. Although women are at greater risk for macular degeneration than men, smoking, high cholesterol, and genetic predisposition may also contribute to the disease, which is usually brought on by age.

Macular degeneration affects about 5% of people over 65, but the risk is about 30% for those over 75. In 1997, $75 million was allocated by the National Institutes of Health specifically to study the disease.

Results

This test produces images of the inside and back of the eye, particularly the veins, which are illuminated by the dye. Blood flow in the eye and the retina can be observed. Circulatory disorders as well as retinal detachment or degeneration is visible. This test is often used to assess and monitor diabetic retinopathy.

The prevalence of cataract increases with age. In persons, aged 55-64 years, one study found 33% of the respondents with early cataract and 6% with late cataract. In persons over 75 years, these figures were 37% and 52%. The frequency of visually significant cataract is lower in men than in women. "Early cataracts" are those that cause no symptoms. "Late cataracts" cause symptoms or have functional significance.

Electroretinogram (ERG)

This sophisticated test observes the functioning of rods, cones, and the optic nerve.

Procedure

After numbing and dilation (or widening) of the pupils, electrodes are placed on the head of the reclining patient. Contact lenses wired to electrodes are inserted in the eyes. The electrodes measure eye movement and response to a series of light flashes and patterns shown in a darkened room. Because the eyelids are held open, this test is disconcerting and uncomfortable. However, the eyes stay moist with drops administered by the doctor or technicians.

Results

By measuring response to light, this test diagnoses nerve damage or other malfunctioning within the eye. Deviations from normal response can indicate such damage.

A-Scan (Ocular Biometry)

If a patient has been diagnosed with cataracts and surgery is necessary to replace the lens, this test is performed.

Ophthalmologists are physicians who spend two to four additional years studying the eyes after they graduate from both college and medical school. They can write prescriptions for eyeglasses, contacts, and drugs, as well as perform necessary tests, procedures, and surgeries.

Optometrists are Doctors of Optometry who examine, diagnose, treat and manage diseases and disorders of the visual system. They are empowered to write prescriptions for eyeglasses and contact lenses, low vision aids, visual therapy, and a limited range of drugs to treat eye diseases. They may also perform certain surgical procedures.

Opticians are trained according to state regulations to fabricate, fit and adjust eyeglasses and contact lenses. They are authorized to instruct patients in the proper use of eyeglasses and contact lenses. However, in order to provide eyeglasses or contact lenses for a client, they must first have a prescription from an ophthalmologist or optometrist.

Procedure
The eyes are dilated, and a light shined into the eye measures the power of the current lens.

Results
Using computer technology, the shape, thickness and power of the eye's natural lens is determined, so that a plastic replica with the same focusing properties can be made and placed in the eye during cataract surgery.

Corneal Topography and Corneal Pachymetry
These tests are used to determine the patient's eligibility for laser vision correction and to diagnose corneal disease.

Procedure
During a pre-surgery exam, sophisticated equipment is used to take measurements of the cornea's thickness and map the curvature of the eye's surface.

Results
If topography reveals an irregular-shaped cornea or pachymetry finds a too-thin cornea, you may be rejected for laser surgery.

A few tests not listed here may be performed on the eye. Most of these are non-location specific tests which are widely diagnostic. Information on these tests can be found elsewhere in the book or in the terms section. These tests include: MRI, PET and X-ray,

For Further Information

National Eye Institute
2020 Vision Place
Bethesda, MD 20892-3655
(301) 496-5248
www.nei.nih.gov

American Optometric Association
243 Lindbergh Boulevard
St. Louis, MO 63141
(314) 991-4100
www.aoanet.org

American Academy of
Ophthalmology
655 Beach Street
Box 7424
San Francisco, CA 94109-7424
(415) 561-8500
www.eyenet.org

EAR, NOSE & THROAT

The Ear, Nose and Throat (ENT) specialty is called Otorhinolaryngology—oto for ear; rhino for nose; and the larynx is the voice box area of the throat. An otorhinolaryngologist spends fours years studying this specialty after graduation from both college and medical school.

These areas offer opportunities for doctors to obtain indications of general health in addition to information about a specific organ.

As with other senses, many disorders and diseases of the ears and nose are age-related, and should be tested for more frequently as we age. Some of the common complaints in these areas include hearing loss, vertigo (dizziness), and tinnitus (ringing in the ears). Sinus problems, congestion, post-nasal drip and difficulty with swallowing are noted often as well. The exposure of the ears, nose, and throat to the outside world makes them quite susceptible to infection. There is a modern class of antibiotics called aminogly-cosides, which include drugs such as gentamycin and tobramycin, that may cause damage to both the hearing and balance functions of the inner ear, as well as to the kidney. Surprisingly, the most common ear toxin is aspirin: large doses cause tinnitus or ringing.

THE TOP 6 SIGNS OF HEARING LOSS

? Mistaking words in conversation or missing notes at a concert.

? Not realizing that the doorbell or phone has been ringing.

? Suspecting friends and relatives of mumbling intentionally.

? Withdrawal from social situations if frustrated with hearing.

? Constant ringing or hissing in the background.

? Some sounds are very loud and annoying.

The most common form of hearing impairment in people between adolescence and age fifty, especially for the estimated 5 million Americans with occupational exposure to hazardous noise levels, is noise-induced hearing loss. Hearing can be damaged by one intense, loud noise, or by constant exposure, such as that in a factory. Noises above 90 decibels, such as a jet plane, a rock concert, or a jackhammer, are all risks for hearing damage. The ear can often adjust to loud noises, but unexpected noise can cause irreparable damage. Only rarely, though, does an eardrum actually rupture.

The human sense of smell usually functions in tandem with the sense of taste. However, the nose is approximately 10,000 times more sensitive than the tongue. When your nose is blocked, you lose nearly 90% of the taste sensations.

The thyroid gland, located at the front of the throat, produces the hormones which control the body's metabolism and energy use. The thyroid is an endocrine gland which produces hormones that are carried throughout the body by the blood stream. Thyroid dysfunction affects 1% to 4% of adults in the United States. Thyroid diseases, such as hypothyroidism (the thyroid does not produce enough hormones, making the body sluggish), hyperthyroidism (the opposite of hypothyroidism, making the body agitated), and thyroid cancer, are more common among women than men. Goiter, an enlarged thyroid, is often visible as a swelling of the neck. The thyroid is such a source of medical difficulty for some people that they may be referred to an endocrinologist for diagnosis and treatment. Tests of the thyroid are usually ordered when symptoms of its malfunction are observed elsewhere in the body.

THE TESTS

EARS

Audiometry (Hearing Test)

Audiometry tests a patient's range of hearing.

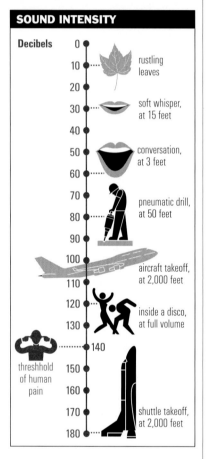

SOUND INTENSITY

Decibels	
0	
10	rustling leaves
20	
30	soft whisper, at 15 feet
40	
50	conversation, at 3 feet
60	
70	pneumatic drill, at 50 feet
80	
90	
100	aircraft takeoff, at 2,000 feet
110	
120	inside a disco, at full volume
130	
140	
150	threshhold of human pain
160	
170	shuttle takeoff, at 2,000 feet
180	

Procedure

In a soundproof room, the patient is usually asked to listen to sounds with and without headphones. A technician pipes tones of different pitches into speakers in the room or into the head-phones. The patient is asked to indicate when a tone is heard, and whether it is heard in the right or left ear. By varying the pitch of the tone, the hearing range or the nature and extent of hearing loss can be determined.

Results

The test looks for hearing damage due to trauma or deterioration over time. A hearing aid may be recommended if hearing is found to be damaged.

> Prolonged ringing of the ears or pain from sound are indications of severe hearing damage. As a person goes deaf, the high tones generally go first, then speech becomes both difficult to understand and construct. Eventually, the low tones disappear as well.
>
> The prevalence of hearing impairment increases after age 50. Hearing loss can be identified in over 33% of persons aged 65 years and older, and in up to half of persons over 85 years. Older persons with hearing impairment are particularly prone to problems such as social and emotional isolation, clinical depression, and limited activity. Many people of all ages suffer from hearing problems. It is also a natural part of the of the aging process.

Auditory Brainstem Response

This test checks the effectiveness of the nervous system in relationship to the ears, and may be utilized in the event of certain types of hearing loss, or if tumors are suspected in the inner ear.

Procedure

The patient's head is hooked up to four electrodes and she is asked to lie down in a darkened room with a set of headphones. A series of tones and clicks is played through the head-phones, which often induces sleep in people taking this test. This is normal; the test is measuring the response of the brain to these sounds.

> Only 10% of those who could be helped by hearing aids actually wear them. Hearing aid technology has advanced rapidly in recent years, and very small models are available. Telephones and theaters have also designed audio broadcast systems which new hearing aids can pick up.

Results

This test is important because abnormal electrical responses to these simple noises may indicate a tumor in the brain or ear areas. Hearing loss can also be measured with this test.

Electronystagmogram (Caloric Study, ENG)

This test uses different diagnostic tools to study a variety of neurological problems associated with the ears and eyes.

HOW BALANCE IS ACHIEVED

cochlea

cerebellum

The motion of fluid in **three semicircular canals** connected to the cochlea (in the inner ear) registers the slightest movement of the head. The cerebellum processes this information, together with input from the eyes and receptors in the body.

Procedure

Electrodes are attached to the patient's face, just under each eye and on the bridge of the nose. After the room is darkened, the patient is asked to follow a series of light flashes along a wall. The electrodes record electrical impulses corresponding to eye movement as the lights flash. After that, water, first cold, then warm, is poured into the ears. This stimulates involuntary eye movement (nystagmus). The electrical impulses produced and the movements recorded test the vestibular system of the inner ear, which controls the sense of balance and dizziness. This part of the test may cause nausea and vomiting, because it disturbs the balance centers of the body. There could be problems for patients wearing pacemakers or those with perforated tympanic membranes or those with ventilating tubes in place (for these patients, air is used instead of water).

Nystagmus refers to involuntary rapid movements of the eye in response to certain stimuli. Often these are the result of an abnormality in the balance mechanism of the body, controlled by the inner ear. Usually done on patients who complain of dizziness, this test evaluates the likelihood of a tumor or infection.

Results

Electrical charges caused by eye movement are picked up by electrodes placed near the eyes and recorded on a graph for analysis. Any abnormalities in movement of the eyes or the electrical impulses can be traced to hearing loss, vertigo, or nerve damage, possibly due to brain damage, inflammation or cancer.

5 TOP SUGGESTIONS FOR THOSE WITH HEARING LOSS

1 Consult a doctor.

2 Avoid situations with a lot of background noise.

3 Tell others you have trouble hearing, not to shout, and ask them to repeat or reword what you don't understand.

4 Ask about the availability of amplification earphones at theaters and public events.

5 Always look at the person speaking to you. Even people with normal hearing interpret information from lip movements and facial expressions.

Tympanogram

This test assesses the movement of the tympanic membrane (or eardrum).

more tests

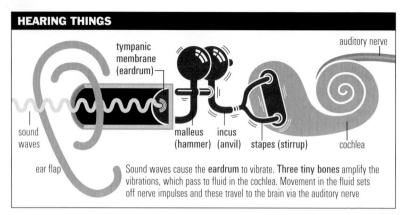

HEARING THINGS

tympanic membrane (eardrum)

auditory nerve

sound waves

ear flap

malleus (hammer)　incus (anvil)　stapes (stirrup)

cochlea

Sound waves cause the **eardrum** to vibrate. **Three tiny bones** amplify the vibrations, which pass to fluid in the cochlea. Movement in the fluid sets off nerve impulses and these travel to the brain via the auditory nerve

Procedure

As in audiometry above, the patient dons headphones. However, these headphones come equipped with a rubber plug, which fits into the ear and up against the eardrum. Pressure is exerted on the plug to test the elasticity of the membrane, which is then recorded by a graphing machine.

Results

Flexibility of the membrane is directly related to its ability to accurately convey sound to the brain. If the graph indicates an abnormal reaction to pressure, it may be the sign of infections, fluid trapped inside the ear, or a perforated eardrum.

NOSE

HOW WE SMELL

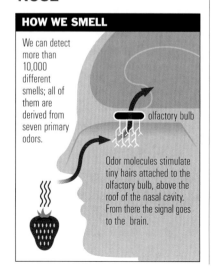

We can detect more than 10,000 different smells; all of them are derived from seven primary odors.

olfactory bulb

Odor molecules stimulate tiny hairs attached to the olfactory bulb, above the roof of the nasal cavity. From there the signal goes to the brain.

Aspiration and Excisional Biopsies

These tests are the beginning of the diagnostic process for serious problems of the sinus.

frontal sinus

ethmoidal cells

maxillary sinus

sphenoid sinus

Procedure

These two procedures investigate the sinuses. Both involve a local anesthetic administered to the mouth or nose tissue. In the first, a needle is inserted through the nose and into the sinuses, where it can remove tissue or fluid samples. In the second, tissue samples themselves are cut away from the sinus area. These samples are taken for further examination, such as cultures, blood tests, studies for cancer, etc. There is discomfort involved in having the instruments inserted into the nose and the slight pain of breaking the skin in the sinus area. Bleeding and discomfort may continue for a few days after the tests.

Results

Tests performed on sinus tissue can reveal sinus infections, tumors of the mouth and sinus cavity, as well as many other problems. *See biopsy in the Terms section.*

Allergies result when the immune system overreacts to exposure to a chemical or natural substance. Asthma and hay fever are examples of such allergies. Many allergens are inhaled. Pollen from grass and trees irritates the nose and sinuses, causing runny nose and tearing eyes. Dust and pet shedding can also cause these reactions.

THROAT

Laryngoscopy

This test is a type of endoscopy (*defined in Terms section*) in which the throat is examined for general health or blockage problems.

Procedure

This test is performed under local anesthesia with a laryngoscope, a flexible, tubular instrument about ten inches long. The scope is a complex instrument, and includes fiber optic visualization equipment, a light source and biopsy equipment. Before the test begins, the mouth and throat are anesthetized with a spray. The laryngoscope is inserted either through a nostril or directly into the throat via the mouth. This is slightly uncomfortable, and despite the anesthesia often produces the urge to gag.

Results

The visualization equipment of the scope can show doctors or technicians infections or tumors of the throat and allow a general internal inspection. Other instruments on the scope allow for fluid or tissue collection from the throat area. These samples can be analyzed in a lab for infection and cancerous cells.

Throat Culture

This is a laboratory test of a swab from the throat that is cultured to investigate infection.

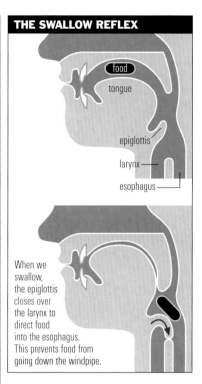

THE SWALLOW REFLEX

food

tongue

epiglottis

larynx

esophagus

When we swallow, the epiglottis closes over the larynx to direct food into the esophagus. This prevents food from going down the windpipe.

Procedure

A technician inserts a cotton swab deep into the mouth and throat, producing a gag reflex.

This transfers potentially infected mucus and saliva onto the swab, which is then rubbed onto a culture plate. If infection is present, the fluid will grow more bacteria.

Results

This test searches for infection. Growth of certain kinds of bacteria on the culture over a period of time indicates to the doctor that an infection is present, and usually results in the prescription of antibiotics.

Streptococci should be identified in throat cultures, because a specific type of streptococcal pharyngitis (i.e., beta-hemolytic) may be followed by rheumatic heart disease or glomerulonephritis (inflammation of the filtering units of the kidney).

Excisional Throat Biopsy

This type of biopsy removes a tissue sample from the throat in order to test for infected tissues or tumors.

Procedure

This test may be performed in a doctor's office or in a hospital, but it is always performed under general anesthesia. Once the patient is under anesthesia, the doctor has better access to areas deep in the throat. Using surgical tools, a small tissue sample is removed for biopsy. Once awakened from the anesthesia, the patient may experience soreness and bleeding in the throat for several days. Because of the general anesthesia, the patient should not drive home from the test. This test can take several hours to be performed, and a patient should plan on spending the better part of a day.

Results

The biopsy of the throat seeks infected tissue, or, more likely, tumors or other growths. The biopsy attempts to determine their nature and severity in order to help doctors decide how to proceed. A serious cancer may require surgery and further treatment; a benign cyst may simply be removed.

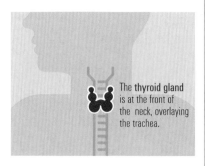

The thyroid gland is at the front of the neck, overlaying the trachea.

Thyroid Stimulating Hormone (TSH) Blood Test

The function of the thyroid is governed by several chemicals in the body, levels of which can be used to predict disease.

Procedure

Blood is drawn from a vein in the arm and subsequently sent to a laboratory to be analyzed.

Results

The presence and quantity of TSH and another hormone, thyroxine, can indicate the beginnings of hypo and hyperthyroidism at levels undetectable in other types of exams.

Radioactive Iodine Uptake (RAI)

This test studies the thyroid's ability to manufacture hormones.

Procedure

After the iodine is administered either orally or intravenously, the patient is asked to lie down on an examination table. Once the iodine has spread through the body, radioactive pictures of the thyroid area are taken over a period of several hours. A gamma camera measures the differences in radiation in various parts of the thyroid, much like a Geiger counter. This test is dangerous to those who are allergic to iodine and shellfish. Since the level of radioactivity is low in the chemicals being used, there is little risk of dangerous exposure.

Results

Iodine is a chemical absorbed almost exclusively by the thyroid, and one which shows up well on these nuclear scans. The pictures measure absorption over time, showing the thyroid's functioning ability. Too much or too little indicates that the thyroid is under- or overactive. This means it may be malfunctioning in its regulation of the metabolism.

Thyroid Radioisotope Scan

This thyroid function test is similar to the one described above.

Procedure

After receiving a radioactive substance (usually orally), the patient lies down on an x-ray table, neck stretched out by a brace. The scanner passes over the patient multiple times and takes pictures of the thyroid area. Unlike the iodine test described above, this not an absorption test over time. Rather, the substance absorbed makes the thyroid stand out clearly in the x-ray pictures. There is no pain involved in this test, and very little radiation risk, as the exposure is very low.

Results

The test is used to evaluate nodules (lumps) in the thyroid. This test may indicate the likelihood of the nodule being benign (harmless) or malignant (cancerous).

> TMJ stands for temporomandibular joint, the part of the jaw which connects to the head at the ear. TMJ dysfunction is used to describe chronic pain associated with this joint. This pain can be associated with chewing, grinding of teeth, or other jaw motions. TMJ dysfunction is being diagnosed more and more frequently in the US. Its exact causes and cure are unknown, though many treatments, both invasive and noninvasive, are evolving. Diagnosis is made through a combination of patients' descriptions of symptoms and physical examinations.

For further information

American Academy of
Otolaryngology
One Prince Street
Alexandria, VA 22314
(703) 836-4444

American Tinnitus Association
P.O. Box 5
Portland, OR 97207
(800) 634-8978

Thyroid Foundation of America
(800) 832-8321
www.clark.net/pub/tfa

Self Help for Hard of Hearing
People, Inc.
7910 Woodmont Avenue
Suite 1200
Bethesda, MD 20814
(301) 657-2248

Every
20 seconds,
a person in the
United States
has a heart
attack.

The heart is the muscular pump that beats continuously from before you are born to your last day of life.

It expands and contracts at the rate of 100,000 beats per day, and pumps about 2,000 gallons of blood every twenty-four hours. During an average lifetime, the heart contracts more than 2.5 billion times. Heart tests may be ordered by your primary care physician, or you may be referred to a cardiologist, who specializes in diseases of the heart. **More is known about gender differences involving the heart than any other organ, yet such differentiation is not always recognized in medical diagnostic testing.**

Men's hearts, although larger than women's, beat more slowly, even during sleep.

Advances in the prevention and treatment of heart disease over the past fifty years have been extraordinary, and deaths due to coronary artery disease have decreased 34%.

THE TOP 5 QUESTIONS TO ASK YOUR DOCTOR ABOUT HEART TESTS

Is this test a routine screening test, or do you see symptoms that cause you to suspect heart disease?

Is there a less invasive test that can provide you with the same information about my heart?

What are the possible courses of treatment if the tests indicate evidence of heart disease?

If the results of my test suggest heart problems, should I be prepared for a hospital stay or surgery?

What are the risks involved in the particular test being recommended? Radiation? Allergy to dyes? Bleeding? Possible heart attack?

Unfortunately, coronary artery disease is still the number one killer of American

women. One in ten American women 45 to 64 years of age has some form of heart disease, and this increases to one in five women over 65. Cardiovascular diseases claim more female lives every year than the next 16 causes of death combined, and almost twice as many as all forms of cancer. **More than 250,000 women each year die of coronary heart disease, compared to 46,000 deaths from breast cancer.** Scientists have found that women who smoked fewer than ten cigarettes daily had a 30% higher risk of death from heart disease or lung disease than women who did not smoke. For women who smoke ten cigarettes or more a day, the risk skyrockets to 80%.

New and emerging technologies for treatment of coronary problems, such as external counter-pulsation, transmyocardial laser revascularization, thrombolytic drugs, and the minimally invasive coronary artery bypass surgical techniques (PortCAB, the Octopus system, or the MIDCAB system) are beyond the scope of this book on diagnostics. However, you should consult with your doctor in order to assure that you have the benefit of the latest technology for treatment.

THE TOP 5 WAYS TO REDUCE THE RISK OF HEART DISEASE

- Quit smoking.
- Cut back on foods high in fat, saturated fat and cholesterol.
- Monitor and manage blood pressure and cholesterol levels.
- Exercise regularly at aerobic levels.
- Maintain normal weight for your height.

THE TESTS

Electrocardiogram (EKG or ECG)

The heart is regulated by electricity. Electrical pulses stimulate the beats of the heart. These pulses, which should be regular in terms of rhythm and frequency, are measured in this test to determine the health of the heart muscle and to identify abnormalities of heart rhythm or rate.

UNDERSTANDING EKG or ECG

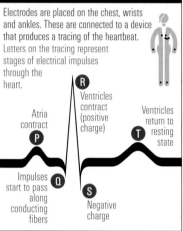

Electrodes are placed on the chest, wrists and ankles. These are connected to a device that produces a tracing of the heartbeat. Letters on the tracing represent stages of electrical impulses through the heart.

R Ventricles contract (positive charge)

Atria contract **P**

Ventricles return to resting state **T**

Impulses start to pass along conducting fibers **Q**

S Negative charge

Procedure

This test is usually ordered when any symptoms of heart disease—such as chest pain—present themselves, and may be part of a normal physical for patients over certain ages. The patient disrobes from the waist up and lies down. Electrodes are attached to the wrists and ankles with gel. One larger electrode is placed on the chest. This is moved around to different spots near the heart during the test. The test lasts about 15 minutes as the 5 electrodes take amplified readings of the heart's electrical activity. There is no risk of being shocked, and the test is entirely painless.

Results

The results, a 12-line graph, are studied by the doctor. This graph gives a picture of how the heart is working, and can reveal the presence of abnormal rhythms, heart inflammation, and

heart disease. It is an extremely safe, painless diagnostic test, but it gives no indication as to whether a heart attack is imminent. It is, however, useful to compare electrocardiograms done at different times on the same patient, because it can identify warning signs.

Several variations of this test exist. One, called the Holter Monitor, is a 24-hour EKG, which measures the heart throughout an entire day, watching for changes which occur when the body is sleeping, digesting, or moving around, and looking for broader patterns in heart rhythm. Another is called an exercise stress test. During this test, the electrodes are attached as during other EKGs or ECGs, but the patient exercises on a treadmill instead of lying down. This gives readings showing the response of the heart to physical exercise. Additional problems can be detected this way, and this test is often done before a more invasive coronary angiograph with cardiac catheterization is performed.

AN EXERCISE STRESS TEST

Electrodes are placed on the chest, and a blood pressure cuff is wrapped around the arm.

EKG, heart rate and blood pressure readings are taken as you exercise slowly on a treadmill (or stationary bicycle.)

Chest X-Ray

This plain x-ray can identify many problems in general, although specific information about the heart is often sought. It searches for abnormal heart size or lung congestion (heart failure),

ANATOMY OF A HEARTBEAT

In a cycle that repeats about 70 times a minute, heart muscles pump blood through the heart into the body.

1 Diastole

Atria and ventricles dilate; blood flows into them.

left atrium

right atrium

right ventricle

left ventricle

2 Atrial systole

The atria contract, pushing any remaining blood into the ventricles.

3 Ventricular systole

The ventricles contract, sending blood from the heart to the lungs and the rest of the body.

closed valve

open valves

lung problems (pneumonia, blood clot, tumors) and rib cage abnormalities (cancer, broken bones) in the upper chest.

Procedure

The patient undresses from the waist up and stands next to the x-ray plate. A lead screen may be provided to cover the genitalia to protect them from exposure to radiation. The x-ray camera is aimed at the chest and the pictures taken. The film is then removed from the x-ray plate to be developed, which takes only a short while. To evaluate the heart, a frontal and side view are usually obtained.

Results

The heart, lungs and ribs are all visible in this type of x-ray. Broken or otherwise abnormal ribs can be seen, as can large tumors, clots or fluid in the lungs. Emphysema can also be diagnosed based on the results. Abnormal heart size or shape may be seen as well.

Echocardiogram

This ultrasound test can give an accurate picture of the structure and inner workings of the heart in motion with considerable accuracy and without the radiation of an x-ray.

Procedure

The patient lies down on a table, removes clothing from the waist up, and a gel is spread on the chest which will help transmit sound waves. The transducer, the pen-like instrument used in all ultrasounds, is passed over the heart area of the chest until a good spot can be found. The technician moves the transducer around the heart area for approximately half an hour, taking readings.

Results

The sound waves bouncing from the transducer to the body and back can be converted into both pictures and graphs. The pictures are like a video of the inside of the heart as it beats. The doctor can determined the internal size of the heart chamber, the thickness of the chamber walls, whether there is excess fluid building up around the heart, contractile power of the heart muscle, and whether the four valves of the heart are narrowed, inflamed or leaking. The main value of an echocardiogram is in identifying abnormalities of heart valves, and in calculating a number called the "ejection fraction," which is useful in diagnosing heart failure. The "ejection fraction"is the percent of blood in the heart that is pumped out with a single beat.

more tests ▶▶

Coronary Angiography with Cardiac Catheterization

An angiogram is a specialized x-ray which is done by injecting radiopaque dye (a radioactive substance) into the blood vessels leading to the heart in order to visualize abnormalities (narrowing of the arteries). Structural abnormalities in the heart absorb the dye at different rates, and thus the x-rays identify these structures. While angiography is used in blood vessels outside the heart, it is particularly useful with the heart and the blood vessels through which it pumps blood.

Cardiac catheterization is one of the greatest advances in cardiology in recent medical history. It is a test that is performed when coronary artery disease is suspected, and is used to decide whether or not surgery is necessary.

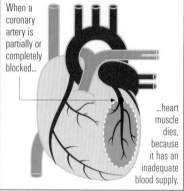

BLOCKED BLOOD SUPPLY

When a coronary artery is partially or completely blocked...

...heart muscle dies, because it has an inadequate blood supply.

Procedure

The test is done in a special room, usually in a hospital, and requires a fair amount of preparation by the patient, including fasting from the previous night and taking a sedative. Electrocardiogram (EKG or ECG) monitors will be attached to the patient to measure heart rate and rhythm while the test is going on. A thin catheter is inserted into a vein or artery of the body, usually in the upper leg/groin area, after this area

has been anesthetized with an injection. The catheter is guided through the body into the heart itself. The catheter can also be used to take pressure readings, collect blood, and inject dye into the heart. (Less commonly, dye is simply injected into a blood vessel.) As the dye spreads through the body to the area of interest (specific blood vessels or the heart) x-rays are taken of that area. Although an important diagnostic tool, this procedure does involve risk. Approximately 1 in 1000 patients die of a heart attack during or after the procedure. However, the risk of dying from a cardiac event for high risk patients is much greater than the risk of death during the procedure.

Results

This test is usually performed following an EKG or ECG, Echocardiogram and stress test. The doctor can clearly see clogged arteries or malfunctioning heart tissue with this test, both at the end of the catheter and through the x-rays that can be obtained. This can lead the doctor to decide about bypass surgery, angioplasty, revascularization procedures or drug therapy.

Nuclear Heart Scans: Thallium, Stress-Thallium, Technetium

The nuclear scan is important in diagnosing heart disease. It can measure the health of heart tissues, as well as provide images of heart function.

Procedure

One of several nuclear isotopes is injected into the body. All isotopes are absorbed differently as the blood moves through the heart, depending on damage to it. Shortly after injection, the gamma camera is used to photograph the heart.

Results

The pictures from this test can detect whether areas of heart tissue have died during a heart attack. The doctor can also see if some areas of the heart are not getting sufficient oxygen or are not pumping properly. This often causes the painful condition known as angina. The doctor may order additional tests, such as angiography with cardiac catheterization after seeing these results. This test replaces the exercise stress test in patients for whom exercise poses great risk.

Electron Beam Computed Tomography (EBCT) or Ultrafast CT

This relatively new noninvasive test is able to accurately determine the amount of calcium content in coronary arteries, which some medical experts believe may be a predictor of heart disease.

Procedure

Utilizing a specialized type of Ultrafast CT scanner with electron beams, the patient is asked to lie on a large tray which slides into the scanner. The scan may require twenty to thirty minutes, during which the patient is requested to lie still. The procedure is entirely painless, but will expose the patient to higher levels of radiation than a normal x-ray series, although well within medically acceptable limits.

Results

Because this electron beam technique allows the technicians to take higher speed images, they can capture x-ray pictures of the moving vessels as the heart is beating. EBCT scanning is promising as a preventive tool because the test is painless, noninvasive, and risk free. However, it is considered a controversial emerging technology with a high rate of false positive and negative results. Also, experts disagree about whether or not calcium deposits in the arteries are accurate predictors of future risk of coronary artery disease.

SIGNS OF HEART DISEASE

- Chest discomfort,
- Shortness of breath,
- Fatigue and
- Palpitations and
- Dizziness.

RISK FACTORS INCLUDE

- Hypertension
- Diabetes
- Elevated cholesterol
- Smoking
- Obesity
- Lack of physical activity.

Blood tests for lipids/cholesterol, triglycerides, HDL, LDL

Lipid is a term for any fat in the bloodstream. Excess buildup of lipids can clog arteries and cause heart attacks and strokes. Blood tests for lipids evaluate risk of heart disease, clogged arteries, diabetes and pancreatitis (in the case of triglycerides). Taken over time, they also measure the effect of exercise on fat in the blood.

Procedure

Blood is drawn after the patient has been fasting, and is sent to a lab for analysis.

Results

Many measurements return from a lipid test. Cholesterol is a fatty compound which is produced in the body and is necessary in small quantities, but can build up and clog arteries when blood levels are high. Triglycerides are the most dominant lipid in the body, and have some correlation to heart disease. Low Density Lipoprotein (LDL) is often referred to as the "bad"or dangerous cholesterol product. High Density

more tests

Lipoprotein (HDL) is the beneficial or "good" cholesterol, and has an inverse relationship to heart disease: high HDL decreases the risk. LDL is the opposite: high LDL increases the risk of heart disease.

Apolipoproteins Blood Test

Apolipoproteins—the protein fractions of lipoprotein molecules—are an important component of the blood. They may indicate the patient's risk of coronary artery disease.

Procedure

Blood is taken from a vein and sent to a lab for analysis.

Results

High levels of the lipoprotein are indicative of potential risk of coronary artery disease, among other illnesses.

Blood Test for Heart Enzyme, CPK (creatine phosphokinase), CK (creatine kinase), SGOT (serum glutamic-oxaloacetic transaminase), LDH (lactate dehydrogenase)

These are all substances which exist in muscle, including heart muscle, and leak into the blood when a heart attack or other damage has occurred. Elevated levels in the bloodstream can indicate such damage. This test often accompanies an EKG test in order to diagnose heart attacks.

Procedure

Blood is drawn from a vein and sent to a lab for analysis. Sometimes this test is done immediately after a patient is admitted with chest pain, so the circumstances may vary.

Results

If elevated levels of CPK, LDH or CK are found in the bloodstream, they may have come from damaged heart, brain or muscle cells. More specific tests can

be done to localize these enzymes, which leak for up to two days after a heart attack.

SGOT is found in both the liver and the heart, and is always found in measurable amounts in the bloodstream.

No one of these enzymes is definitive evidence of heart damage, but they are examined in conjunction with an EKG to assist in diagnosis. These tests are sometimes repeated over several hours to determine if an evolving pattern of muscle damage can be identified.

Blood Test for Vitamin B1

A poor diet can result in vitamin deficiencies. Although this test is not specific to or diagnostic of heart disease, a lack of vitamin B1 can be particularly dangerous to the heart.

Procedure

Blood is drawn from a vein and sent to a lab for analysis. Fasting is required before the tests so that vitamin-rich foods do not adversely affect the outcome.

Results

A low level of the vitamin, usually due to poor diet, can lead to muscle weakness and potentially to heart failure. If found, vitamin deficiency is usually treated with vitamin supplements.

Hematocrit Blood Test

This general blood test measures red blood cells as a percentage of total blood volume in a sample (see Complete Blood Count), but this test is not specific to or diagnostic of heart disease.

Procedure

Blood is drawn from a vein or from a finger prick for analysis. The hematocrit is simply the measure of the height of the column of red blood cells after a blood sample goes through a centrifuge, which separates blood into its parts.

Results
A low reading can indicate anemia, while an abnormally high reading can mean poor oxygenation of the blood, which occurs commonly in certain kinds of congenital heart disease and in emphysema.

Blood Test for Antimyocardial Antibodies
Some chemicals within the body are confined within an organ unless the organ is damaged. At that point, these compounds leak into the bloodstream or urine.

Procedure
Blood is drawn from a vein and taken to a lab for analysis.

Results
These antibodies may be present in the blood in cases of rheumatic heart disease or certain kinds of weakness of the heart muscle.

For Further Information:

American Heart Association
7272 Greenville Avenue
Dallas, TX 75231
214-373-6300
www.americanheart.org

Center for Cardiovascular Education
www.heartinfo.org

One out of 28 women aged 60 develops breast cancer.

One out of 41 women aged 50 develops breast cancer.

One out of 2,500 women aged 20 or less develops breast cancer.

BREASTS

The primary function of the female breast is to provide milk for nursing infants, but the breast is also a secondary sexual characteristic that has been regarded by society as a symbol of femininity, beauty, and eroticism. It consists of fifteen to twenty lobes of milk-secreting glands that are embedded in fatty tissue. During pregnancy, estrogen and progesterone stimulate the milk-producing glands and cause the nipple to enlarge for feeding.

The doctor who specializes in the health of the breast is the same specialist who cares for other female reproductive organs, a gynecologist. There are specialists within obstetrics and gynecology, such as obstetricians, who deal with pregnancy, and gynecological oncologists, who deal with cancer of the female reproductive system, including breast cancer. Surgery for breast cancer is usually performed by a general surgeon, while medication treatment of breast cancer may be performed by a medical oncologist.

Although women periodically have breast problems such as non-cancerous tumors and minor infections, **the most serious medical problem concerning the breast is cancer. Having an immediate family member develop breast cancer makes it much more likely that a woman will develop it.** A number of other predisposing factors have been identified, including obesity, early onset of menstruation, and delayed or absent child bearing. Like other cancers related to female genitalia, prolonged exposure to estrogen may increase the risks. Tamoxifen is a prescription that blocks estrogen and can dramatically reduce breast cancer risk. Unfortunately, it is associated with increased risk of uterine cancer. Other drugs with similar effects are available or under development.

Breast cancer may occur in men as well as women, but is much more common in women. **A total of 180,000 new cases are detected annually, and the disease caused approximately 44,000 deaths in 1997.** One in 8 or 9 American women contracts breast cancer at some point in life, and the likelihood of developing the disease increases with age — 80% of breast cancers occur in women over the age of fifty.

As is true of cervical cancer, **early detection is the key to isolating and stopping breast cancer.** All women should inspect their breasts monthly (see diagram on page 56). Although most breast cancers (70%) are self-detected, a mammogram is one of the best ways for women to protect themselves against breast cancer. Women over 40 should have a mammogram every other year; women over 50 should have one annually.

THE TOP 6 QUESTIONS TO ASK YOUR DOCTOR ABOUT YOUR BREASTS

- If I think I have a problem with my breasts, what should I do right away?
- What is the best test to diagnose my particular symptoms?
- Are there any conditions (such as pregnancy) that would make a particular test a bad idea?
- Are there any restrictions on my diet or activities before the test?
- Does the clinic or hospital require a patient consent form in order to take this test?
- How will I feel after the test?

THE
TESTS

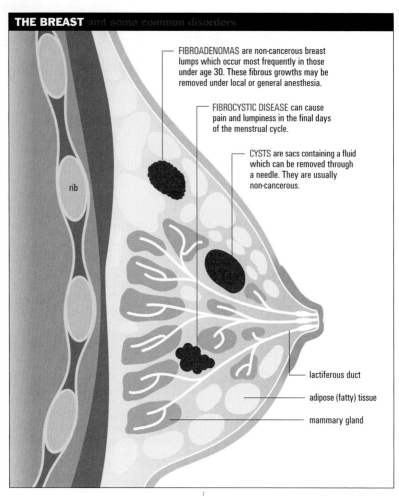

THE BREAST and some common disorders

FIBROADENOMAS are non-cancerous breast lumps which occur most frequently in those under age 30. These fibrous growths may be removed under local or general anesthesia.

FIBROCYSTIC DISEASE can cause pain and lumpiness in the final days of the menstrual cycle.

CYSTS are sacs containing a fluid which can be removed through a needle. They are usually non-cancerous.

rib

lactiferous duct

adipose (fatty) tissue

mammary gland

Mammogram

This important test is an x-ray of breast tissue. Mammography can detect a lump up to two years before it can be felt by manual examination.

Mammograms can fail to detect cancer up to 10% of the time. Large breasts, or those made up more of ducts and fibrous tissue than fat (this occurs in 70% of women 40 and older) can hide small tumors. Ultrasound is being used more often in women who have breasts that render the mammogram less effective.

Procedure

The test may be done lying down, sitting or standing. The breasts are x-rayed, one at a time. The woman places one breast between two plates which compact the breast and spread it out. The x-ray machine, attached to the plate, then takes a picture. The procedure is repeated with the other breast. This procedure is, at best, uncomfortable and embarrassing. At worst, it can be painful. Communicate to your doctor or technician your level of discomfort and request reasonable adjustments.

Results

The pictures of the breast show fat and duct tissue in the breast. Tumors as well as duct tissue will stand out from the breast tissue. If a tumor is suspected from a mammogram, a biopsy will likely be performed.

A lumpectomy is a procedure to surgically remove a tumor from the breast. More serious is the mastectomy procedure, which removes the entire breast. Cosmetic and reconstructive surgery is now able to replace lost tissue and retain the original shape and form of the breast. This may also improve the patient's health. Chemotherapy is also a common treatment in addition to surgery.

MAMMOGRAM

1 A breast is placed on the top of the x-ray table, and is pushed down by a plastic cover.

2 An x-ray is made of each breast in turn.

3 If a tumor is present, it will appear as a dense mass on the x-ray film.

Thermography

This is an alternative technique for diagnosing breast cancer, not requiring x-ray radiation. It measures heat in the breast using an infrared camera. However, it is not as precise as a mammogram.

Procedure

Like in a mammogram, the woman places each breast in turn between two plates, spreading each out. The infrared camera then photographs the breast. This camera is sensitive to heat.

Results

Areas which are hotter than others receive more than normal blood flow. Therefore, if an area shows up "hot" on the infrared camera, it can be suspected to be tumorous, and a biopsy can be ordered.

Tumor Marker Blood Tests, Cancer Antigen (CA) Blood Tests

A number of blood tests have been discovered which can detect cancers in very specific parts of the body, notably in the breast, and can also be used to monitor the spread of cancers and the effectiveness of treatment.

Procedure

Blood is drawn from a vein and sent to a lab for analysis.

Results

Though these tests can be used to detect and monitor cancer, particularly breast and ovarian cancer, they also pick up on benign tumors and, sometimes, cirrhosis of the liver. Though they may be improved as genetic technology advances, currently only the first wave of tests are available.

Breast biopsies are performed on all suspicious tissue. Previously, this was done with an invasive procedure that required injections and surgery under general anesthesia. Now it is most often done by inserting one needle into the breast and withdrawing tissue through the needle.

If breast cancer is detected, the lymph nodes in the armpits are usually the first area to be considered for surgery, since cancer can be ferried to other parts of the body by the nodes. Using a radioactive dye process, however, doctors can now pinpoint which lymph nodes will be affected by breast cancer and remove only those, sparing the patient pain and the difficulty of being without the nodes.

TEST YOURSELF (once a month, 2 or 3 days after the end of your period)

1 IN THE SHOWER, raise your left arm. With the fingers of the right hand, carefully examine the left breast. In a circular pattern, starting from the outer top, press firmly enough to feel the tissue inside the breast. Complete one full circle, then move toward the center and circle again. Continue until you reach the nipple.

Check the area above the breast, including the armpit, for lumps.

Repeat the examination on your right breast.

2 IN FRONT OF A MIRROR, place your hands at your sides and check your breasts for any changes in color, shape, or size. Also look for any dimpling or scaling of the skin.

3 STILL IN FRONT OF THE MIRROR, place your hands on your hips. Press your shoulders and elbows forward to flex the chest muscles.

Then raise your hands and clasp them behind your head. Check for everything in step 2.

4 LIE DOWN, and place a pillow under your left shoulder. Raise your left arm above your head. Using the circular method from step 1, examine your left breast.

Repeat the process for your right breast.

FINALLY, gently squeeze each nipple to check for discharge. Report any changes to your doctor.

 A Clinical Breast Examination (CBE) is essentially the same procedure as the self-exam, except it is performed more thoroughly by a doctor, who has more expertise, and who may use the CBE as an opportunity to educate patients in techniques for their self-exams.

For Further Information:

Y-Me National Organization for
Breast Cancer
Information and Support
212 Van Buren
Chicago, IL 60607
312-986-8228 or 1-800-221-2141

National Alliance of Breast Cancer
Organizations
2nd Floor
1180 Avenue of the Americas
New York, NY 10036
212-719-0154

The Breast Cancer Information
Clearinghouse
www.nysernet.org/breast/Default.html

The Mayo Clinic Breast Cancer
Decision-making Guidelines
www.mayohealth.org/mayo/9907/htm/
breastcan.htm

U.S. Department of Health and
Human Services
Breast Cancer and Mammography
www.oncology.medscape.com/govmt/
DHHS/patient/DHHS.BreastCancer.
html

La Leche League International
9616 Minneapolis Ave.
Franklin Park, IL 60131
1-800-LA-LECHE (1-800-525-3243)

Fanlight Productions Breast
Reconstruction
47 Halifax Street
Boston, MA 02130
617-524-0980

Breast Implant Information Line
Food and Drug Administration
1-800-532-4440

LUNGS

The lungs are the main organ of the respiratory system. They supply the body with oxygen (O_2) and eliminate carbon dioxide (CO_2). Some tests on the lungs may be ordered by your personal physician. You may be referred to a pulmonologist, a doctor with several years of specialized training in diseases of the lungs. These diseases may be acute (many resulting from an immediate condition such as pneumonia) or chronic, having to do with exposure to a given problem over time (such as emphysema from cigarette smoke).

Lung disease is the number three cause of death in the United States, responsible for one in every seven deaths.

THE TOP 6 QUESTIONS TO ASK YOUR DOCTOR ABOUT LUNG TESTS

If I have a problem breathing, what should I do right away?

What is the best test to diagnose my particular symptoms?

Are there any conditions that would make a test a bad idea?

Are there any restrictions on my diet or activities before the test?

Does the clinic or hospital require a patient consent form in order to take this test?

How will I feel after the test?

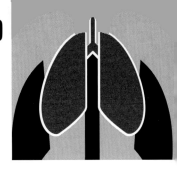

More women die from lung cancer than from any other type of cancer, including breast cancer, and cigarette smoking is the primary cause. In 1999, lung cancer claimed an estimated 68,000 women, compared with 43,300 female deaths from breast cancer.

A woman's lungs are more susceptible than a man's to tobacco exposure **Women who smoke are approximately ten times more likely to develop lung cancer than nonsmoking women.** Tobacco use is also a major risk factor for other cancers, such as cervical and esophageal (food pipe) and throat cancer, as well as other respiratory problems such as emphysema and chronic bronchitis. A woman who smokes is two to six times more likely to suffer a heart attack than a nonsmoking woman, and the risk increases with the number of cigarettes smoked each day. Unfortunately, approximately 22.5 million American women are smokers.

Asthma, an important lung condition, affects approximately 5% of the population. Between the ages of 20 to 50, women outnumber men 3 to 1 in asthma-related hospital admissions. Although the basic cause of asthma is not yet understood, there is evidence that it may be related to women's hormonal changes during menstruation or pregnancy.

THE TESTS

Arterial blood gases

This blood test is not performed routinely. For patients with potentially more serious lung conditions, it measures levels of oxygen, carbon dioxide, and acid in the blood in order to determine lung function. Abnormal levels of the various gases may indicate the lungs are failing to bring oxygen in and expel CO_2 properly, suggesting lung disease.

Procedure

Because this test is slightly more difficult than other blood tests, blood must be obtained from an artery rather than from a vein. Arteries are usually found deeper in the arm than veins. The blood sample is then sent to a lab for analysis. This test is often performed on patients whose lung function is in question, or before surgery.

Results

Lung disease and heart disease often go hand-in-hand. The lung's function is to remove CO_2 and put oxygen into the blood. The heart's job is to pump the blood to the entire body, where oxygen is delivered to tissues and CO_2 is picked up for expulsion. Blood gases by themselves are not indicators of specific diseases. However, abnormal blood gas levels are an important indicator of how well the heart and lungs are functioning, and can provide important information in making a diagnosis.

Carboxyhemoglobin

Acute carbon monoxide exposure is often deadly. In addition, long-term exposure at low levels, which can occur at factories or in some homes, can cause serious medical problems. The carboxyhemoglobin test is a measure of carbon monoxide in the blood, which can be used to explain symptoms.

Procedure

Blood is drawn from a vein and sent to a lab for analysis. This test is not done very often, but may be ordered for women who complain of fatigue and headache which are suspected to be environment-related.

Results

The result is expressed in a percentage of carboxyhemoglobin in the blood. Carbon monoxide attaches or bonds to hemoglobin (the oxygen-carrying pigment found in red blood cells), preventing it from carrying oxygen, which is why it is so dangerous. If more than 5% of hemoglobin is found to have carbon monoxide, it is likely that some external factor is contributing the gas to the body.

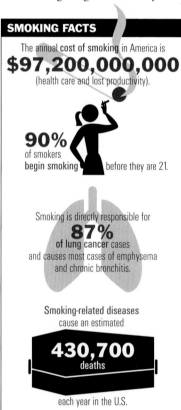

SMOKING FACTS

The annual cost of smoking in America is

$97,200,000,000

(health care and lost productivity).

90%
of smokers begin smoking before they are 21.

Smoking is directly responsible for
87%
of lung cancer cases and causes most cases of emphysema and chronic bronchitis.

Smoking-related diseases cause an estimated

430,700
deaths

each year in the U.S.

Pulmonary Function Test (PFT or Spirometry)

Lungs constantly inflate and deflate as we breathe. There are many measures of the "mechanics" of breathing.

When abnormal, these can point to certain diagnoses. Examples of these measures include how much air is taken in with one breath, how fast it can be expelled and how much is left after letting the breath out.

Procedure

This test simply involves breathing down a tube into a machine which measures lung capacity and strength. The patient is given a mouthpiece attached to a machine and is instructed to breathe into it normally, inhale or exhale deeply, or perform similar tasks.

Results

The results of this test are measured on an instrument called a spirogram. Results can be used to diagnose diseases such as asthma and emphysema, or to see how these diseases are affecting breathing ability.

Bronchogram

Although this x-ray is not needed frequently, it is designed to get a clearer picture of the lungs than a normal chest x-ray can provide.

Procedure

This test requires a considerable amount of patient preparation, including fasting and taking both a sedative as well as a medication to decrease mucus production. The mouth is also anesthetized or "numbed" with a spray or swab, and anesthetic drops are placed deeper into the throat. A plastic tube called a catheter is inserted through the mouth into the lungs. Contrast material (which shows up on an x-ray) is injected into the lungs through the catheter, where the progress of breathing distributes it throughout the lungs. X-rays are then taken of the lungs. This test often induces a lot of coughing.

Results

The contrast material outlines the airway tubes, and shows up on an x-ray. The appearance of the x-rays can help make a diagnosis.

Bronchoscopy

This is a type of endoscopy that uses a special camera that can go around narrow passages in order to actually look directly at the tissues inside the bronchial tubes. It can also be used to remove an object lodged in the windpipe or to take a biopsy.

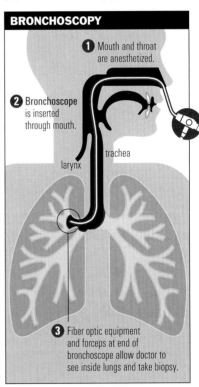

BRONCHOSCOPY

① Mouth and throat are anesthetized.

② Bronchoscope is inserted through mouth.

trachea

larynx

③ Fiber optic equipment and forceps at end of bronchoscope allow doctor to see inside lungs and take biopsy.

Procedure

As with the bronchogram, the mouth and throat are anesthetized. The patient takes a sedative and is given other medication to decrease secretions. The bronchoscope, a flexible tube, is inserted through the mouth, down the windpipe and into the bronchial tubes. At the end is fiber optic visualization equipment and biopsy equipment. A biopsy can be obtained with forceps that actually cut a piece of tissue, or with a brush that gathers cells for collection. This

more tests

test sometimes involves a certain degree of discomfort and anxiety. (That is why a sedative is given.) The patient should arrange to be driven home after this test. The test provides a pulmonologist with the most direct information possible about the condition of the tissues.

Results

Sometimes an x-ray of the bronchial tubes and lungs cannot not reveal small problems. This test allows the doctor to look directly into the area and observe closely any tumors, clots or foreign objects lodged in these areas. Biopsies can be performed on the tissue and blood and fluid samples can also be taken. This procedure is primarily used to diagnose tumors.

ASTHMA

An estimated 14.6 million persons in the United States have asthma, a condition marked by coughing and difficulty in breathing. An asthma attack, which can be triggered by smoke, pet hair, pollen or other allergies, respiratory infections, exercise or strong odors, is a narrowing or thickening of the bronchial tubes which lead to the lungs. Its cause is not understood, but several types of treatment can control most asthma attacks effectively. Still, 5,600 American people die of asthma every year. Approximately 33% of asthma patients are under the age of 18. It is the most common chronic illness among children.

Mediastinoscopy

This endoscopy is performed less often than bronchoscopy. It is performed through an incision in the chest. Rather than examining the lungs directly, a scope called a mediastinoscope is used to directly examine the lymph nodes and other tissue which surround the lungs.

Procedure

A mediastinoscopy is performed under general anesthesia. The patient is put to sleep in an operating room, and an incision is made in the notch at the top of the ribcage. The endoscope is inserted and can withdraw fluid, allow visualizations, or obtain tissue samples, including lymph nodes. This test involves some risk, as does any procedure under general anesthesia.

Results

While this test draws fluid and can take pictures just as other endoscopies, it is usually ordered to get a biopsy of lymph node tissue. Doctors may suspect cancer of the lymph nodes or lungs, which can be detected with a biopsy. Some other diseases of the lung, such as tuberculosis, can also be diagnosed through this procedure.

Sputum culture

Sputum is the name given to any material that is expelled from the lungs. Thus, it is more than just saliva and mucus. This material is tested for evidence of infection by being cultured for bacteria, tuberculosis or other organisms.

Procedure

The patient coughs up sputum into a cup, which is taken to a lab for analysis. A mist which promotes coughing may be administered to stimulate production of sputum.

Results

An analysis of sputum can help diagnose pneumonia and bronchitis and, most importantly, tuberculosis.

Influenza and pneumonia combined are the sixth leading cause of death in the United States.

Thoracentesis

The lungs sit in what is called the "chest cavity." Sometimes abnormal amounts of fluid can collect in the small space between the lungs and the chest cavity wall. A thoracentesis withdraws this fluid from the chest for analysis.

THORACENTESIS

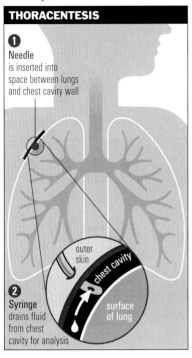

❶ Needle is inserted into space between lungs and chest cavity wall

outer skin

chest cavity

surface of lung

❷ Syringe drains fluid from chest cavity for analysis

Procedure
A small area of the chest is injected with a local anesthetic. Then, a needle is inserted and is positioned into the space where the fluid has collected. Fluid is removed with a syringe for analysis. If needed, a larger amount can be drained if it is causing discomfort or intruding on normal body functions such as breathing. This test can be performed in the doctor's office and should last not more than approximately 30 minutes. The patient should arrange to be driven home after this test.

Results
The analysis from the lab reports on the content of the fluid. This can include protein, glucose, bacteria, and cancerous cells. Fluid around the lungs can indicate lung cancer and pneumonia, as well as other chest abnormalities or infections.

Lung scan
There are two types of this nuclear scan, which tests for blood clots in the lung, abnormal oxygen absorption and lung function.

Procedure
In the first type of test, a radioactive substance is injected into a vein and spreads to the lungs. A "gamma camera" then takes pictures of the lungs. In the second type, the patient inhales a gas containing radioisotopes into the lungs and pictures are then taken. The radioisotope is not dangerous in the small amount given.

Results
The radioactive substance injected into the vein will not spread to areas of the lung where blood vessels are blocked by blood clots. Thus, areas with clots will not show up on the nuclear scan pictures. The pictures from the gas test demonstrate which parts of the lung are effectively exchanging air. If the gas does not absorb into some parts of the lung, it means those parts are not working properly. Both types of lung scan, together called a "ventilation-perfusion" lung scan, are most commonly performed in patients in whom a blood clot is suspected.

For Further Information

The American Lung Association
432 Park Avenue South
8th Floor
New York, NY 10016
1-800-LUNG-USA (1-800-586-4872)
www.lungusa.org

Asthma In America Survey Project
1901 L Street NW
Suite 300
Washington, DC 20036
(202) 452-9429
(202) 296-3727 fax
www.asthmainamerica.com

The liver processes about six cups of blood each minute, extracting nutrients and oxygen.

LIVER

The liver is the largest solid organ in the body.

It weighs between 2.5 and 3.3 pounds and is about the size of a football. It manufactures the majority of chemicals in the body, and regulates the levels of most of the main chemicals in the blood. It converts glucose into material that can be stored and used later. It also breaks down fats and proteins, and produces enzymes necessary for blood clotting. It processes bile, a necessary ingredient to digestion, and filters drugs and alcohol out of the body. Although the liver is quite complex in its functions, it is not delicate. **The liver is so durable that up to 75% of its cells can be destroyed or surgically removed before it ceases to function.** Though it is not fragile, its complexities make it extremely important to the overall function of the body.

Disorders of the liver include hepatitis (liver inflammation), cancer, tumors, cysts, bile duct/gallbladder diseases and cirrhosis. **Cirrhosis** is a name for any of a multitude of chronic diseases which stress the liver and over time cause scarring. Cirrhosis is simply scarring that results from liver damage. Cirrhosis prevents proper blood flow to the liver, so that it cannot continue to produce the proteins and other necessary substances the body needs. It also slows the ability of the liver to process nutrients and toxins. Most commonly associated with alcoholism, cirrhosis is the seventh leading cause of death by disease overall. For Americans between

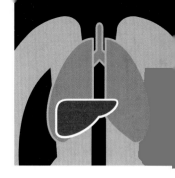

the ages of 25 and 44, it is the fourth largest disease-related cause of death. **Liver disease due to excessive consumption of alcohol outnumbers all other types of liver disorder by five to one.** CT scans can be used to detect cirrhosis and other liver disorders. The liver can also be biopsied.

Hepatitis may be caused by viral infection, alcohol abuse, chemicals, or prescription drugs. Various strains of viral hepatitis from A through G and GB have been identified. All can be damaging to the liver. Hepatitis A and B are preventable with vaccines and controllable. **There are an estimated 3.9 million Americans with Hepatitis C, for which there is no vaccine and no definitive treatment.** (A cocktail of Interferon and Ribavirin has shown promising results in treating Hepatitis C, but this treatment is still being tested.) Liver damage due to Hepatitis C is the leading cause of liver transplants in the United States.

For hepatitis, preventive measures and early detection through testing are the best protection.

THE TOP 5 WAYS TO BE GOOD TO YOUR LIVER

- Don't drink excessive amounts of alcohol.
- Avoid foods high in fats.
- Drink 6 to 8 glasses of water daily.
- Maintain normal weight for your height.
- Maintain abdominal muscle tone.

THE
TESTS

IT'S ABOUT THE SIZE OF A FOOTBALL

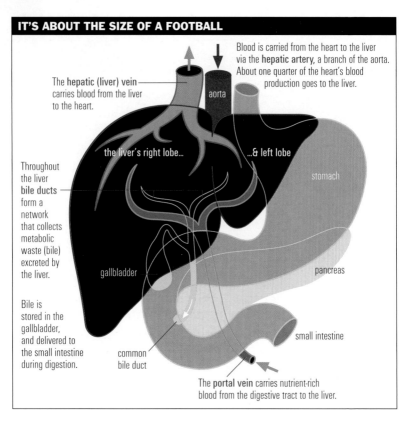

Blood is carried from the heart to the liver via the **hepatic artery**, a branch of the aorta. About one quarter of the heart's blood production goes to the liver.

The **hepatic (liver) vein** carries blood from the liver to the heart.

aorta

the liver's right lobe…

…& left lobe

stomach

Throughout the liver **bile ducts** form a network that collects metabolic waste (bile) excreted by the liver.

gallbladder

pancreas

Bile is stored in the gallbladder, and delivered to the small intestine during digestion.

common bile duct

small intestine

The **portal vein** carries nutrient-rich blood from the digestive tract to the liver.

Endoscopic Retrograde Cholangiopancreatography (ERCP)

The bile ducts connect the liver to the small intestine through a small opening called the ampulla of Vater in order to distribute bile for digestion. An endoscope, inserted via the mouth, examines the liver via this opening, and is particularly useful for taking successful x-rays of the bile ducts in order to determine the presence of cancer, infection, blockage with gallstones, scarring, or some obstruction within the bile duct. Cancer of the pancreas may also be diagnosed with this procedure.

Procedure

The patient fasts for 12 hours before the test, so that the intestine will be as clear as possible. The mouth and throat may be anesthetized, and a sedative is often given as well. The endoscope, about the diameter of a finger, is then inserted through the mouth and guided into the stomach and small intestine. The endoscope can enter the ampulla and usually does so to inject dye into the bile ducts. X-rays are then taken of the liver area, and other endoscopic procedures can be performed. These include removal of stones from the bile duct area. Because of the use of anesthesia and possibly sedatives, the patient should be driven home after this test.

Results

The x-rays of the liver area should be very clear because of the dye injected. Bile duct infections and blockages should be visible. Because the scope allows detailed inspection of this area of the body, other problems or blockages may be revealed. The material removed from the biopsy can be tested for cancers or infections. This test is safer than exploratory surgery and may provide the same result.

Abdominal Ultrasound

This ultrasound can be used to evaluate the liver, aorta, kidney, gallbladder, lymph nodes, uterus and ovaries, and other solid organs in the abdomen. The intestines, however, do not show up well on the ultrasound.

Procedure

The patient disrobes from the waist up and lies down on an examination table. A gel is put on the abdomen to help transmit sound waves. The technician then moves the transducer over the parts of the abdomen which are of importance to the doctor.

Results

Like other ultrasound results, these appear on a screen which can be studied by the doctor. This test reads gallstones and kidney stones especially well. It can detect inflammations and also differentiate between solid and fluid-filled masses, useful for examining suspected tumors. It is helpful in identifying masses outside the liver or gallbladder compressing these organs. Depending on the results of the ultrasound, the doctor may request a biopsy of the organs involved.

Each year, more than 25 million Americans suffer from liver and gallbladder diseases, and more than 43,000 die of liver disease annually.

Computed Tomography of the Biliary Tract and Liver (Liver CT Scan)

Multiple x-ray scans of the biliary tract and liver are reconstructed by computer as two-dimensional images on a monitor. Sometimes a contrast medium is used to accentuate differences in tissue density.

Procedure

The patient is asked to lie down on an x-ray table, and the table is positioned in the opening of a scanning gantry. If a contrast medium is taken orally, the patient may be asked to fast until after the test. If a contrast medium is introduced intravenously, no fasting is necessary. The scanning process can take as long as an hour, during which the patient is requested to remain as motionless as possible.

Ultrasonography is often performed on the liver instead of CT because it is less expensive and does not expose the patient to radiation. The CT scan usually provides a level of detail that ultrasound cannot.

Results

The size, shape and function of the liver can be observed from the CT. Cysts, tumors and abscesses will show up on the CT.

Percutaneous Liver Biopsy

Under local anesthesia, a special hypodermic needle is inserted through the chest wall into the liver, and a sample of tissue is drawn out by aspiration. This sample allows medical specialists to determine the health of the liver tissue.

Procedure

The patient is asked to lie down and to remain as still as possible. An anesthetic is injected, and when the area is sufficiently anesthetized, the patient is asked to take a deep breath, exhale, and hold her breath at the end of the expiration. A special needle with a flange to control depth of penetration, called a Menghini needle is used to penetrate the upper abdominal wall and the liver, and, using the plunger of the syringe, to aspirate a small specimen of tissue into the tip of the needle. This process should take place in a few seconds, but the patient is usually required to remain resting under the doctor's observation for two hours. Under certain circumstances, the needle may require guidance to a particular place in the

more tests ⏩

liver, in which case, CT scanning or ultrasound may be performed simultaneously with the biopsy.

Results

The specimen of tissue must be transported to the laboratory for analysis immediately. Examination of the tissue will reveal signs of cirrhosis, hepatitis, or infections such as tuberculosis. Tissue analysis will also identify various forms of cancer, as well as non-cancerous tumors.

Mono Spot Blood Test

This blood test for mononucleosis, a debilitating illness that swells the liver and spleen, enables the doctor to make a definitive diagnosis. Mono, which often occurs in teenagers and young adults, manifests itself in extreme fatigue, prolonged headache, strong fever and sore throat.

Procedure

Blood is drawn from a vein and sent to a lab for analysis.

Results

If the test comes back positive, another confirming test may be performed.

Alanine Aminotransferase Blood Test (ALT) or Serum Glutamic-Pyruvic Transminase Blood Test (SGPT)

Injury or disease in the liver causes leakage of this enzyme into the bloodstream. The most likely diseases causing this leakage are hepatitis, mononucleosis or acute injury with infection, drugs or alcohol.

Procedure

Blood is drawn from a vein and sent to a lab for analysis.

Results

An elevated level of ALT in the blood is a sign of liver inflammation.

WHY ALCOHOL ABUSE IS BAD FOR YOUR LIVER

1 Most alcohol is converted by enzymes in the liver into **acetaldehyde** which, like alcohol itself, is toxic to liver cells.

inside a single liver cell

2 Acetaldehyde causes **alcoholic hepatitis**, which inflames and damages liver cells and the liver's ability to function.

cell damage

cell damage

3 Alcohol abuse also causes fat to accumulate in liver cells, a condition called **fatty liver**.

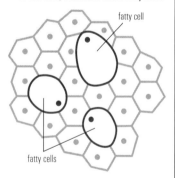

fatty cell

fatty cells

4 If people with alcoholic hepatitis or fatty liver continue to abuse alcohol, **cirrhosis**, which is irreversible, can develop.

In cirrhosis, **scar tissue** forms on the liver, separating cells into clumps.

More than 25,000 Americans die each year from cirrhosis of the liver, the seventh leading cause of death.

Alpha-fetoprotein Blood Test (AFP)

AFP is a protein produced by the fetal liver and yolk sac. Increased levels of AFP may indicate liver tumors.

Procedure

Blood is drawn from a vein and sent to a lab for analysis.

Results

This compound is elevated in the blood of patients with liver and other cancers. It can also be elevated by cirrhosis or chronic active hepatitis.

Alkaline Phosphatase Blood Test (ALP)

Although ALP is found in many tissues, it is particularly concentrated in the liver and the biliary tract epithelium. Detection of this enzyme is important for determining liver and bone disorders.

Procedure

Blood is taken from a vein and sent to a lab for analysis.

Results

Elevated levels of this compound in the bloodstream may indicate cirrhosis, obstruction of the bile duct, or a liver tumor.

Bilirubin Blood Test

Bilirubin results from the breakdown of blood cells by the liver, which then eliminates them from the body via the intestines. Too much bilirubin in the body means that blood cells are not being eliminated properly. This can cause jaundice, a yellowing of the skin.

Procedure

Blood is taken from a vein and sent to a lab for analysis. This test is often done in conjunction with a number of other tests, known as liver function tests.

Results

Excessive red blood cell destruction from disease leads to elevated bilirubin. Blockage of the bile ducts from cancer, gallstones, or scarring can also cause elevated bilirubin.

TYPES OF HEPATITIS

A preventable by vaccine; unpleasant but has no lasting effects

B preventable by vaccine; potentially fatal if untreated; controllable with drugs

C no vaccine; extremely dangerous; no definitive cure or control

D rare; only exists as coinfection with Hepatitis B; accelerates liver damage

E extremely rare in U.S.; no chronic liver disease

F extremely rare in U.S.; not sufficiently studied

G blood borne viral infection; long-term effects unknown

Hepatitis B and C can be transmitted by receiving blood transfusions, but today that is rare. The most common causes now are contaminated drug injections and unprotected sex. The most obvious sign of the disease is jaundice, a yellowing of the skin.

Protein, Albumin, Serum Protein, Globulin and Serum Electrophoresis Blood Tests

These proteins are essential to the liver's function as the body's "factory."

Procedure

Blood is drawn from a vein and sent to a lab for analysis.

more tests

Results

Serum protein is high in patients with cirrhosis and leukemia. Low albumin is a sign of kidney disease, edema or fluid in the lungs. Decreased levels of the other proteins are signs of malnutrition, starvation, liver disease, or cancer.

Hepatitis Blood Test

Viral hepatitis, caused by a damaging virus, is the second most common problem with the liver, behind alcoholic liver disease. Hepatitis A is transmitted by eating uncooked food or drinking unsanitary water. It is quite contagious, inflames the liver, and also causes fatigue and muscle aches, but does no permanent damage to the liver. Hepatitis B and C, however, are spread through contact with contaminated blood and are much more dangerous, often leading to cirrhosis or other liver failure. Both B and C also can be transmitted sexually (see also Reproductive Organs).

Procedure

Blood is drawn from a vein and sent to a lab for analysis.

Results

Blood can be tested for the presence of the virus or antibodies to it. Since there is a vaccine for A and B, these antibodies can result in a false positive test. Hepatitis can only be controlled, not cured, with drugs.

Ammonia Level Blood and Urine Test

Ammonia is generated by bacteria acting on proteins present in the digestive system. It then moves to the liver, where it is normally converted into urea and then secreted through the kidneys.

Procedure

A blood sample is taken from a vein and sent to a lab for analysis. If a urine test is required as well, a urine sample is gathered.

Results

Ammonia is always present in blood and urine, but in high quantities indicate severe liver disease.

For Further Information

American Liver Foundation
75 Maiden Lane, Suite #603
New York, NY 10038
1-800-GO LIVER (1-800-465-4837)
www.gi.ucsf.edu/ALF/

National Network for Organ Sharing
1100 Boulders Parkway, Suite #500
P.O. Box 13770
Richmond, VA 23225-8770
1-804-330-8500

American Association for the Study
of Liver Diseases
www.hepar-sfgh.ucsf.edu

Johns Hopkins Division of Infectious
Diseases: Hepatitis
www.hopkins-id.edu/diseases/
hepatitis

American Gastrointestinal
Association
www.gastro.org

National Center for Infectious
Diseases (CDC): Viral Hepatitis
1-888-4-HEP-CDC (1-888-443-7232)
www.cdc.gov/ncidod/diseases/
hepatitis/index.htm

The kidneys filter approximately 40 gallons of blood daily.

Each kidney
is about
4 inches long
(the size shown here)
and weighs
6 ounces.

KIDNEYS

The kidneys, ureter, bladder, and urethra comprise the urinary tract. Kidneys remove liquid waste from the blood in the form of urine, keep a stable balance of salts and other substances in the blood, regulate blood pressure, and produce erythroprotein, a hormone that aids in the formation of red blood cells. **A nephrologist is a specialist who deals with diseases of the kidneys.** Depending on the nature of the complaint or test ordered, a patient may also be referred to **a urologist, who treats problems with the urinary tract once urine has left the kidneys.**

Within the kidney, microscopic units called nephrons filter waste products from the blood.

The efficiency of the kidney diminishes with age as the number of functional nephrons declines. Kidney disorders include kidney cancer, congenital disorders, glomerulonephritis (an inflammation of the nephrons), and kidney stones. Diabetes

and high blood pressure are also common causes of kidney damage.

Kidney stones are one of the most common disorders of the urinary tract, and are extremely painful. Blood in the urine is a frequent sign. Although kidney stones occur more frequently in men than in women, the number of women who get kidney stones has been increasing over the last 10 years. They develop from crystals, usually made largely of calcium, which form in the urine. Approximately 10% of all Americans will develop a kidney stone, although most pass out of the body without a doctor's intervention. **Kidney stones strike people most often between the ages of 20 and 40.** However, once a person gets more than one stone, he is more likely to develop others. Kidney stones are usually detected through urinalysis, which can be confirmed with an x-ray called pyelography.

The ureters carry urine from the kidney to the bladder for storage. Disorders of the bladder include tumors (malignant or benign), disturbance of bladder control (incontinence), which may be due to another illness such as diabetes or multiple sclerosis, and cystitis. Cystitis, an infection, is also known as painful bladder syndrome and frequency-urgency-dysuria syndrome. **About 90% of cystitis patients are women, approximately one-third of whom are over fifty.** Women are more susceptible to cystitis because the female urethra is shorter than the male urethra and this provides less of a barrier to bacteria.

FACTS ABOUT THE KIDNEYS

- More than 20 million Americans are affected by kidney and urologic diseases.

- Renal cell carcinoma, the most common form of kidney cancer, usually occurs after the age of 40 and affects twice as many men as women.

- Kidney disease can occur from taking large quantities of painkillers over many years.

- Women can live in fine health with one kidney. Kidney transplant surgery, however, is not uncommon and is successful in about 80% of all cases.

THE
TESTS

THE URINARY TRACT

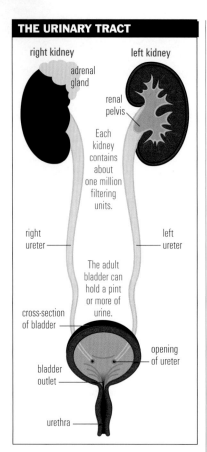

right kidney

left kidney

adrenal gland

renal pelvis

Each kidney contains about one million filtering units.

right ureter

left ureter

The adult bladder can hold a pint or more of urine.

cross-section of bladder

opening of ureter

bladder outlet

urethra

including those taken for kidney disease, can flush electrolytes out of the body and cause dehydration.

Magnesium

Along with calcium and phosphorus, magnesium levels in the body can be abnormal in liver disease and kidney failure.

Procedure

Blood is taken from a vein and sent to a lab for analysis.

Results

Magnesium is largely regulated by the kidney. Too little magnesium in the blood is common in liver disease. Too much is usually a sign of overconsumption, such as taking too much antacid. People with kidney failure have too much magnesium because their kidneys cannot get rid of it.

> Magnesium is essential in the formation of bones and teeth, for muscle contraction, and for the transmission of nerve impulses. Found in most foods, it is used in many laxatives as well. Taking too much antacid, particularly in cases of kidney disease, can be very harmful, even deadly.

Electrolytes

These compounds must remain in balance in the blood for survival. They are electrically charged minerals naturally found in the body. Four are usually studied: Bicarbonate maintains the body's acid-base balance. Potassium, sodium, and chloride help maintain the body's fluid balance. This test is almost always done at any suspicion of kidney disease, and on every patient who enters the hospital.

Procedure

Blood is drawn from a vein and sent to a lab for analysis.

Results

Testing for their presence is also a test of dehydration, but can be indicative of problems elsewhere. Any diuretic,

Osmolality

Osmolality measures the concentration of dissolved particles in the blood. It evaluates fluid and electrolyte imbalance in the blood and urine. This test is done when the doctor suspects seizures and dehydration.

Procedure

Blood is taken from a vein and sent to a lab for analysis.

Results

Since the kidney is responsible for maintaining these levels, an imbalance may be a sign of kidney disease.

Phosphorus

Most phosphorus in the body is stored in the bones, and helps regulate calcium levels in the body.

Procedure

Blood is taken from a vein and sent to a lab for analysis.

Results

Along with calcium and magnesium, the amount of this substance in the blood can be used to predict kidney failure. Low amounts of calcium and magnesium usually means lots of phosphorus. This condition indicates kidney and liver failure, and thyroid problems too.

> Phosphorus exists outside the body in two forms, yellow and red. Red cannot be absorbed by the body and is nontoxic. Yellow, on the other hand, is readily absorbed and very toxic. It is found in factories, fireworks, and some rat poisons.

Sodium

Sodium is one of the most important minerals in the body. The kidney and brain work together to find a sodium balance. If too much sodium—in the form of table salt—is ingested, the brain will tell the kidney to flush more out of the system.

Procedure

Blood is taken from a vein and sent to a lab for analysis.

Results

Excess sodium building up in the body may be an indicator of kidney failure or malfunction. Diminished sodium in the body is clinically more common than levels which are too high.

Blood Urea Nitrogen (BUN), Creatinine, Creatinine Clearance

These tests are usually done together in a "panel" with the the previous three, and are almost always performed when any kidney trouble is suspected. The kidneys usually filter urea nitrogen and creatinine out of the body.

Procedure

Blood is taken from a vein and sent to a lab for analysis. The creatinine clearance test measures the amount of creatinine in both blood and urine over time, so samples of both are taken over the course of a day.

Results

Presence of too much urea nitrogen or creatinine in the blood is an indication of kidney failure. The creatinine clearance test measures exactly how well the kidney is functioning by checking how much of the waste product is removed, and how fast. This gives doctors important beginning information and can lead to further investigation. Too little BUN in the blood may be an indication of liver problems or of malnutrition.

Urinalysis

This common test evaluates urine based on a number of factors. It can lead to a diagnosis of a huge number of diseases, or merely indicate general health. Because urine is so readily available and any abnormality in the body often causes some abnormality in the urine, this test is universal.

Procedure

The patient urinates into a sample cup which is then sent to a lab for analysis. The urine is then analyzed for color, appearance and odor. The pH (acidity) is taken. A small amount can be cultured to test for bacteria. Some is examined under a microscope, looking for abnormal particles or blood in the urine. Any sediment in the urine can be analyzed and its content determined. Dipsticks, pieces of plastic coated with chemicals that change color in the presence

more tests

of other chemicals, can be dipped into the urine to test for these chemicals.

Results

Though many tests can be done during a urinalysis, several are always done. The urine is examined visually, and cloudiness or blood indicates a problem. The specific gravity, which measures the volume of particles dissolved in the urine, can alert doctors to kidney problems. A low or high pH can be a sign of kidney failure, infection, diabetes or dehydration. The presence of glucose in the urine indicates diabetes or other kidney problems. Ketones in the urine indicate diabetes or starvation. Nitrite in the urine is a good indication of infection. Protein in the urine usually means the kidney filters have been damaged.

Urine Amino Acid Screen

Usually, only small amounts of amino acids are found in urine. More than a small amount can indicate kidney problems.

Procedure

The patient urinates into a sterile container, which is then sent to a lab for analysis.

Results

An increase of amino acids in urine means that the kidney is not handling them properly, a sign of disease.

Urine Culture

Normal urine is sterile. It contains fluids, salts, and waste products, but is free of bacteria, viruses, and fungi. This test cultures urine to see if bacteria grows, indicating a urinary tract infection. It is usually done during urinalysis.

Procedure

The patient urinates into a sterile container, which is then sent to a lab

for analysis.

Results

Bacteria in the urine is a sign of a urinary tract infection. Antibiotics are usually given to treat the infection.

Urinary tract infections are more common in women than in men, and may be caused by sexual activity or by organisms that have spread from the rectum, bladder or kidneys. They are not uncommon in women who have been hospitalized with a catheter. Careful personal hygiene, drinking plenty of fluids, and regular emptying of the bladder can prevent these infections.

24 Hour Urine (Steroids, calcium and protein)

Since many chemicals in the body fluctuate with food and exercise, looking at one urine sample is often not enough. This tests urine collected over the course of an entire day, every single time the patient urinates.

Procedure

The patient urinates into a sterile container, which is then sent to a lab for analysis. All urine for an entire day is collected for study. The same container is used all day.

Results

The urine is tested for several components. Too much calcium in the urine can be a sign that kidney stones will form or that hormone regulation is damaged. The 24 hour test for protein provides more detailed information about why protein would be in the urine than a standard urinalysis. Uric acid is found in the urine of patients with gout and leukemia, and can contribute to kidney stones as well. Excessive amounts of steroids, produced by the genital organs or other endocrine glands (adrenal glands), can indicate diseases in these organs, such as abnormal menstruation and infertility.

Abdominal X-ray

This test is often the first step in diagnosing abdominal pain. It examines the internal organs of the abdomen, searching for intestinal blockages and tears, tumors and other deposits such as kidney and gallstones (see x-ray under Medical Terms). This test reveals clear pictures of the kidney and bladder, but different, more specialized tests may be required to view the intestines.

Procedure

The patient dons a hospital gown and two x-ray pictures are taken, one lying down and one standing. It is a short and painless test.

Results

Calcium deposits in the kidney and bladder are revealed with this test. If a tumor has blocked the operation of an organ, the backup, not the tumor itself, is visible. Swollen organs are visible, however.

Cystography, Cystourethrogram

Liquid comes to the bladder from the kidney via the ureters, and passes out of the body through the urethra. This test can trace this process with x-rays. The pyelogram may also be conducted for similar purposes. This test is often ordered after an abnormal urinalysis.

Procedure

A catheter is inserted via the urethra into the bladder. The catheter drains any liquid out of the bladder, then injects dye into the bladder. X-rays are then taken.

Results

This test studies the function of the bladder, looking for malfunctions or tumors. If liquid passes back up the ureters toward the kidney, this will be evident on the x-ray. If it leaks out of the bladder, this indicates a tear.

Incontinence is a term for involuntary urination. Approximately 3 million older Americans suffer with this problem, but men are affected less often than women. It can be caused by infections, stones or tumors. Urinalysis and pyelogram can often detect these problems or other blockages.

Pyelogram

This procedure evaluates kidney function. Kidneys often do not show up well on a standard x-ray, so this procedure, involving a contrast dye, is used.

This test is often ordered after an abnormal urinalysis in order to see the flow of blood in the system more clearly.

Procedure

Before this test is performed, it is common to give the patient a laxative to clear the intestine of material which could interfere with the x-ray. A dye is usually injected intravenously, and the patient then waits for it to spread through the blood to the kidneys. X-rays are taken once, the patient urinates, and then pictures are taken again.

Results

The size and shape of the kidneys are apparent, and any abnormality is evident. Cancer of the kidney can be seen, as can infections and kidney stones. If the dye does not spread properly in the kidneys, this indicates bad blood flow and possible kidney failure. The ureters and bladder are also made visible as the dye passes into them.

Renal Angiogram

Similar to the pyelogram above, this test evaluates kidney function and blood flow. Unlike the pyelogram, dye is injected more directly. This test is often ordered after an abnormal urinalysis and for diagnosis of high blood pressure or renal tumors.

more tests ▶

Procedure

First, a local anesthetic is injected into the skin near the femoral artery, a large artery in the leg. A catheter is then inserted into this artery, and it is maneuvered up into the body next to the kidney. The catheter then injects a contrast dye directly into the kidney area, and x-rays are taken.

Results

As with the above test, this diagnoses kidney failure, stones, and cancers. It also diagnoses narrowing of the arteries to the kidneys (blood vessel blockages). It is not taken over a period of time.

Cystoscopy

With this type of endoscopy, the endoscope enters the body through the urethra. This procedure allows the urologist direct examination of the urethra and bladder in order to determine the health of the tissues.

Procedure

The cystoscope is a rigid tube inserted into the urethra and up into the bladder. The urethra, the tube through which this scope travels, is anesthetized with an injection beforehand, but the insertion is still painful. A sedative is recommended. The doctor or technician can then look through the tube and perform various tests. Urine, blood or tissue can be sampled. This test provides an advantage over the standard urine test, because it can take urine from either kidney. Dye may also be injected through the scope, and x-rays taken, a procedure called a retrograde pyelogram. This test usually causes a bit of blood in the urine, and urination afterwards is key to avoiding infection.

Results

This test can visually detect problems in the kidneys and especially the bladder. Tumors or other growths are usually clear. Samples removed can be analyzed for cancer and infection, and x-rays obtained are studied as described above in pyelogram. These x-rays usually show the bladder better than a normal pyelogram. Sometimes, the scope can be used to remove stones.

Cystometry

This test is similar to the one described above, but measures bladder function.

Procedure

The patient first urinates to clear the bladder. A catheter is then inserted into the urethra, and different fluids are inserted and drained out of the bladder. The patient must describe any unusual sensations. The bladder is then filled completely with liquid, measuring the bladder's size and pressure. The fluid may be drained from the bladder and replaced with carbon dioxide for further measurements.

Results

This test measures bladder pressure, sensitivity and other functions. Any abnormalities are reported by the patient or the instruments, and usually lead to further testing. This is an extremely uncomfortable and embarrassing–but safe–test. It is common for the patient to request a sedative before the procedure.

Renin Assay, Plasma

When blood pressure falls, the kidneys release renin, which can be measured in the bloodstream.

Procedure

Blood is taken from a vein and sent to a lab for analysis.

Results

The leakage of this kidney-produced enzyme into the bloodstream is an indication of blood vessel blockage in the kidney area or kidney failure.

More than 260,000 Americans depend upon dialysis because of kidney failure. Dialysis is a mechanical technique which replicates the action of the kidneys, removing waste products from the blood. There are two basic methods. One involves the filtering of blood through an artificial kidney machine outside the body. The other inserts a liquid into the abdomen. The liquid absorbs waste products in the body, and is then drained.

Renogram, Renal Scan

This nuclear scan evaluates blood flow to the kidneys as well as their location and structure. It is the nuclear version of the renal angiography.

Procedure

Several radioisotopes are absorbed specifically by the kidney. One of these is injected into a vein, and it moves to the kidneys. The gamma camera then takes pictures of the kidney area.

Results

This test can show kidney failure, hypertension and cancers. Areas which do not absorb the dye suggest tumors, cysts, and non-function.

For Further Information

National Kidney Foundation
30 East 33rd Street
New York, NY 10016
1-800-622-9010
www.kidney.org

National Association for Continence (NAFC)
P.O. Box 8310
Spartanburg, SC 29305-8310
1-800-BLADDER (1-800-252-3337)
www.nafc.org

American Foundation for Urologic Disease
1128 N. Charles Street
Baltimore, MD 21201
1-800-242-2383
www.afud.org

American Urogynecologic Society
2025 M Street NW
Suite 800
Washington, DC 20036
202-367-1167
www.augs.org

GALLBLADDER

The gallbladder is a small pear-shaped sac located under the liver. The purpose of the gallbladder is to concentrate and store bile manufactured by the liver before sending it on to the duodenum, where fat digestion occurs. The gallbladder swells between meals as it fills with bile, then expels it into the digestive tract to help food digest. Gallbladder problems are rare in childhood and early adulthood. **Gallstones** are crystals of cholesterol, bile, and pigment that form in the gallbladder. They may obstruct the passage of bile into the intestinal tract, causing inflammation, and symptoms of pain, nausea, and diarrhea or generalized infection. They cause severe pain in the upper abdomen for up to four hours at a time, frequently after a meal.

Women between the ages of 20 and 60 are twice as likely to develop gallstones as men in this age group. The likelihood of developing gallstones increases for both sexes thereafter. Obesity is a major risk factor for gallstone formation, as is crash dieting and prolonged fasting. About 1 million people are diagnosed with gallstones every year, but many carry *silent* stones, which have no symptoms and are usually not problematic.

Gallstones and kidney stones are not related. The most common test for detection of gallstones is the abdominal ultrasound. This is a painless study performed by bouncing sound waves off of the upper quadrant of the abdomen and photographing the image. Gallbladder testing is usually conducted under the supervision of a gastroenterologist, who specializes in disorders of the digestive system.

& PANCREAS

The pancreas is an elongated carrot-shaped gland that lies along the back of the abdomen, behind the stomach. It consists primarily of exocrine tissue which secretes digestive enzymes and hormones into the body. The enzymes break down carbohydrates, fats, proteins, and nucleic acids in the digestive system. The hormones, insulin and glucagon, regulate the level of glucose in the blood.

Because the pancreas is part of both the digestive and the endocrine systems, pancreatic tests may be ordered under the supervision of either a gastroenterologist or an endocrinologist. Diseases of the pancreas include cystic fibrosis (a genetic disorder that predisposes the patient to long term lung infections and prevents the pancreas from producing enzymes essential to the absorption of fat), pancreatitis (which may result from excessive alcohol intake or from viral infection) and pancreatic cancer. **By far the most common pancreatic disorder is diabetes mellitus,** in which the insulin-producing cells in the gland are damaged or destroyed. Insulin helps the sugar from food get into body cells. If the body doesn't make enough insulin, sugar from food cannot get into the cells. Instead, it stays in the blood, elevating blood sugar levels and keeping the body malnourished and tired.

Diabetes, the sixth leading cause of death among those 65 and older, affects approximately 10% of older women and is a cause of illness and early death. Diabetic patients, especially those in poor metabolic control, are susceptible to a series of long-term small and large blood vessel complications that can affect every aspect of physical function. Limbs may lose feeling, and eyesight is often affected. Older persons frequently underreport symptoms because they curtail their physical activity to avoid the onset of symptoms, or because their physical function is already impaired by other conditions.

Women at risk for Type II diabetes
are over 45
are African-American, American Indian, Latino, or Asian
have a family history of diabetes
are overweight
do not exercise regularly
have low HDL or high triglycerides

Diabetic patients, especially those with poor sugar control, are susceptible to a series of long-term small and large blood vessel complications that can affect every aspect of physical function. Limbs may lose feeling, and eyesight is often affected. Older persons frequently underreport symptoms because they curtail their physical activity to avoid the onset of symptoms, or because their physical function is already impaired by other conditions.

THE
TESTS

THE BILIARY SYSTEM

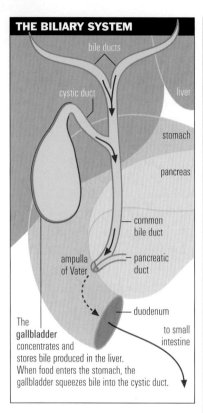

bile ducts

cystic duct

liver

stomach

pancreas

common bile duct

ampulla of Vater

pancreatic duct

duodenum

to small intestine

The gallbladder concentrates and stores bile produced in the liver. When food enters the stomach, the gallbladder squeezes bile into the cystic duct.

GALLBLADDER

Endoscopic Retrograde Cholangiopancreatography (ERCP)

For this test see **LIVER** *page 66*

Oral Cholecystogram

If an ultrasound is unable to make a clear diagnosis of pain in the gallbladder, this test will be ordered. The oral cholecystogram utilizes a contrast dye to highlight the gallbladder.

Procedure

In this test, the patient swallows a capsule containing a contrast dye the evening before the test. These capsules can cause side effects, but this is rare. The dye is digested and makes its way into the bile the liver produces. This bile is then stored in the gallbladder about 12 hours after the pill is taken. The x-rays are then taken.

Results

The dye makes the gallbladder stand out on the x-rays. Blockages, inflammations, gallstones, and, rarely, tumors, should all be visible. Cholescintigraphy (Gallbladder Nuclear Scanning, Hepatobiliary scintigraphy, or HIDA scanning) is a procedure that differs from a cholecystogram in that a radionuclide contrast dye is injected in a vein. The dye is again concentrated into the biliary tract and gamma rays emitted from the bile can be detected by a scintillator. This is a help in the diagnosis for gallbladder inflammation or obstruction.

Percutaneous Transhepatic Cholangiography (PTC)

This test is a different kind of cholangiogram than described under ECRP in the liver section. It is rarely necessary; however, if the dye in the cholecystogram described above does not cause the gallbladder to show up on x-rays, it probably indicates a blockage to the gallbladder. This more invasive test is then performed. Open cholangiograms may be performed during a surgical operation where dye is injected directed into the biliary tracts to make sure that there is no obstruction in this area.

Procedure

The patient is placed on an x-ray table in the radiology department and the abdominal wall or lower chest wall is anesthetized. Using televised fluoroscopic monitoring, a needle is passed through the abdominal wall and into the liver. A biliary branch is located and punctured. When bile is flowing freely into the needle, radiographic dye is injected. The dye passes into the biliary tract. X-rays are then taken. If an obstruction is found, a catheter or stent is left temporarily in the biliary tract to establish drainage and decompression. The patient may feel some discomfort when the needle is introduced, even though the area is anesthetized. This procedure will take approximately one hour. The patient may feel abdominal pain for several hours after the test, and will normally remain under observation for that period.

Results

As above, the dye should make the gallbladder stand out. Blockages, inflammations, and stones should be visible.

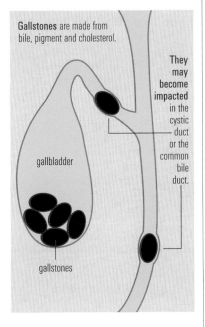

Gallstones are made from bile, pigment and cholesterol.

They may become impacted in the cystic duct or the common bile duct.

gallbladder

gallstones

YOU CAN LIVE WITHOUT A GALLBLADDER

The gallbladder is merely a storage sac which aids in digestion. It is not essential; in fact, some people are born without one. The gallbladder is sometimes removed by a surgical procedure. Each year, more than 500,000 Americans have gallbladder surgery.

A **cholecystectomy** is an operation to remove the gallbladder completely

A **cholecystostomy** opens the gallbladder and removes the stones while leaving the organ itself in place; however, this is rarely done as gallstones may reoccur.

THE TOP 4 WARNING SIGNS OF DIABETES

- Frequent urination.
- Excessive thirst and hunger.
- Family members with diabetes; it often runs in families.
- Sugar binges; diabetes can be detected with blood and urine tests for glucose.

PANCREAS

Amylase

Amylase converts the starch in food into sugar so that it can be used by the body. It is created by the pancreas and salivary glands.

Procedure

Blood is drawn from a vein and sent to a lab for analysis.

Results

If the pancreas or salivary organs are inflamed or damaged, amylase leaks into the bloodstream. Increased presence of this enzyme in the blood indicates these conditions.

C-peptide

This enzyme is in the bloodstream in proportion to insulin, but stays in the body longer, making it a more accurate measure. The blood test for the enzyme is ordered when there is a need to measure insulin.

Procedure

Blood is drawn from a vein and sent to a lab for analysis.

Results

This test is primarily used to monitor insulin in the body, although too much of this enzyme is a sign of renal failure.

Glucose

The body of a diabetic cannot process glucose, the body's blood sugar. This

more tests

blood test measures glucose levels in the body. A variation of the test, called the glucose tolerance test, is ordered on known diabetics. A known (usually large) quantity of glucose is given to the patient to eat, and blood tests are done over time to see how the patient reacts.

Procedure

Blood is drawn from a vein and sent to a lab for analysis. The glucose tolerance test takes both blood and urine samples at half-hour intervals after the meal is eaten.

Results

Too little glucose, hypoglycemia, is a sign of starvation or an overdose of insulin. Symptoms include dizziness and light-headedness. Too much glucose, hyperglycemia, is a strong indication of diabetes.

Insulin allows glucose to be absorbed into the muscle cells and liver, where it can be stored. Hyperglycemia, or high blood sugar, results when not enough insulin is produced to process glucose. Diabetes is defined by the body's inability to produce enough insulin or its ineffective response to insulin. Many diabetics must take insulin shots regularly to process the glucose in their body. If they do not, a coma can result. Hypoglycemia, meaning low blood sugar, results from not eating enough carbohydrates or taking too much insulin or diabetic medication.

Hemoglobin A1C (Glycohemoglobin)

Glucose combines with hemoglobin, a component of blood, to form hemoglobin AlC. This is a storage form of glucose, which stays in the blood long-term and does not fluctuate with meals, as normal glucose would. This test is usually ordered in those who have already had a glucose test which requires further investigation. It monitors the average level of hemoglobin AlC over the ninety days a red blood cell lives.

Diabetes mellitus, the common form of the disease, exists in two types. Type I diabetes usually manifests itself between the ages of 10 and 16. The pancreas suddenly loses its ability to produce insulin. It comes on quickly, and untreated can result in a coma unless the victim injects regularly with insulin. Type II, which is more common, comes on gradually and usually manifests itself after the age of 40.

Diabetes can be controlled. By maintaining blood sugar with insulin injections and/or other medications, a constant weight and healthy lifestyle, it need not greatly alter a person's life. Those who do not monitor the problem, however, can face loss of vision, loss of circulation to the extremities, and pancreatic failure.

Procedure

Blood is drawn from a vein and sent to a lab for analysis.

Results

If high hemoglobin AlC is found as well as high glucose, these factors are a strong indication of diabetes, especially Type II. This test is also used to monitor how well diabetics are controlling their sugar levels with insulin therapy.

Ketones

Ketones, chemical compounds in the blood, exist in high quantities when the body has to burn fat reserves because it is unable to use carbohydrates.

Procedure

Blood is drawn from a vein and sent to a lab for analysis. The patient urinates into a sterile container, which is also sent to a lab.

Results

Both diabetics and people who are

dehydrated or suffering from starvation may exhibit high ketone levels. Ketosis, the accumulation of excessive amounts of Ketones in the body, is usually a medical emergency.

Lipase

The pancreas serves an important function producing digestive enzymes, such as lipase, which digests fats.

Procedure

Blood is drawn from a vein and sent to a lab for analysis.

Results

Elevated levels of this digestive enzyme in the blood occurs when the pancreas is infected or blocked by cysts. This test is less sensitive than the test for amylase, but will detect pancreatic inflammation a longer period of time after the infection occurs.

> Pancreatic cancer is one of the most common cancers in the US. It is difficult to diagnose, and has no direct cause, although smoking and fat-heavy diet may be contributors. It is the fourth most common cancer in men, sixth most common in women (1989). Eighty percent of cases occur in people over 50.

Sweat Test

Patients with cystic fibrosis have high levels of several minerals in their sweat. This disease, which patients are born with, can be treated if detected early.

Procedure

The area to be tested is cleaned and dried. A drug which induces sweat is dropped onto the skin. An electrode is placed on top of the skin, and another on a nearby patch of skin. Low voltage current run between them allows the drug to seep in and sweating begins. The skin is cleaned and dried again, and a piece of absorbent paper is placed on the skin. It absorbs sweat for up to an hour.

Results

The sweat can be tested for the presence of minerals which indicate cystic fibrosis.

> Just as diabetes prevents the pancreas from secreting hormones, cystic fibrosis prevents it from secreting the enzymes necessary for digestion of fats, causing malnutrition. This genetic disorder, which also causes lung damage and infections, is treated with antibiotics and digestive supplements. Untreated, it can be fatal. Cystic fibrosis is the most common inherited disease for Caucasians.

For Further Information

GALLBLADDER

National Digestive Diseases
Information Clearinghouse
2 Information Way
Bethesda, MD 20892-3570
www.nddk.nih.gov/health/digest/
pubs/gallstns

American Gastrointestinal
Association
www.gastro.org/gallstones.html

American Society for
Gastrointestinal Endoscopy (ASGE)
www.asge.org

PANCREAS

The National Pancreas Foundation
P.O. Box 600590
Newtonville, MA 02460
1-877-NPF-FUND (1-877-673-3863)
www.pancreasfoundation.org/

Pancreas.org: An Informational Site
www.pancreas.org

National Institute of Diabetes and
Digestive and Kidney Diseases
Diabetes Prevention Program
www.preventdiabetes.com.

The upper gastrointestinal tract (upper GI) includes the esophagus, stomach and small intestine.

UPPER GI

The stomach is an organ of the digestive system, connected to the esophagus (swallowing tube) above and the duodenum (the first part of the small intestine) below. As any woman who has ever been grateful for stretch-pants after a big meal can attest, the stomach is elastic and expands when food is eaten. In an adult, the average stomach capacity is about 1.5 quarts (or three pints). Because the stomach is also a reservoir, disorders which occur in the process of emptying the contents include tumors, gastritis (inflammation of the stomach lining), and peptic ulcers, the most common serious stomach ailment.

Ulcers occur when stomach acid and other digestive juices attack and break down the stomach or intestinal lining,

and can result from stress, injury or infection. Ulcers are more common after the age of 60. 1 out of every 10 Americans will suffer from peptic ulcers during his or her lifetime, according to the National Institute of Diabetes and Digestive and Kidney Diseases.

THE TOP 5 SIGNS OF STOMACH ULCERS

- Gnawing pain, particularly when the stomach is empty.

- Loss of appetite.

- Excessive gas or vomiting. Vomiting blood or blood in the stool usually means the ulcer is bleeding, a medical emergency.)

- Feeling bloated.

- Weight loss.

The esophagus is the tube which carries food from the mouth to the stomach. Esophagitis is the inflammation of the esophagus — commonly causing the symptom of heartburn. The small intestine is about 21 feet long and it is here that food absorption occurs. Problems with the stomach, esophagus, and small intestine are frequently treated by a gastroenterologist.

A BITE'S PROGRESS: PART ONE

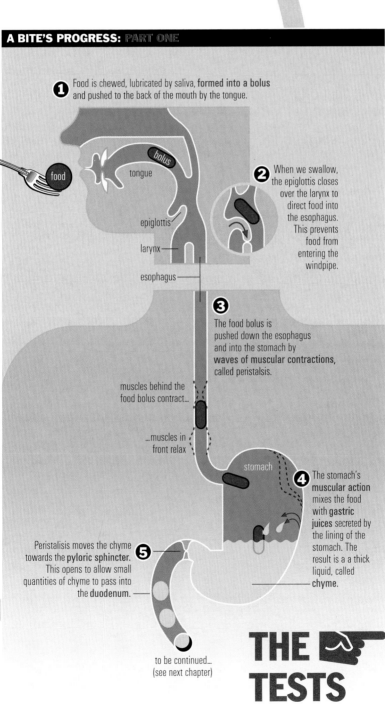

1. Food is chewed, lubricated by saliva, **formed into a bolus** and pushed to the back of the mouth by the tongue.

food

bolus

tongue

epiglottis

larynx

esophagus

2. When we swallow, the epiglottis closes over the larynx to direct food into the esophagus. This prevents food from entering the windpipe.

3. The food bolus is pushed down the esophagus and into the stomach by **waves of muscular contractions,** called peristalsis.

muscles behind the food bolus contract...

...muscles in front relax

stomach

4. The stomach's **muscular action** mixes the food with **gastric juices** secreted by the lining of the stomach. The result is a a thick liquid, called chyme.

5. Peristalisis moves the chyme towards the **pyloric sphincter.** This opens to allow small quantities of chyme to pass into the duodenum.

to be continued...
(see next chapter)

THE 👉
TESTS

ANATOMY OF AN ULCER

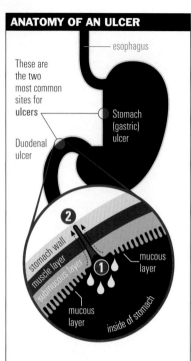

esophagus

These are the two most common sites for ulcers

Stomach (gastric) ulcer

Duodenal ulcer

stomach wall
muscle layer
submucous layer

2

mucous layer

1

mucous layer

inside of stomach

1 The stomach's protective layer of mucous is broken down by increased acid secretion.

2 In time, the ulcer may penetrate all three of the stomach's layers, including the outer wall. This can cause peritonitis.

Gastrin Blood Test

Gastrin is a hormone which stimulates acid secretion and can be measured by a blood test.

Procedure

Blood is drawn from a vein and sent to a lab for analysis. Sometimes injections of substances which stimulate gastrin production are given before the blood sample is taken. This helps determine the cause of high gastrin levels.

Results

Excessive gastrin may indicate tumors (usually in the pancreas). This test is useful in patients with ulcer disease.

Men and women develop gastric ulcers equally. Smoking, drinking alcohol or caffeine, and taking aspirin can irritate an ulcer.

Approximately 20 million Americans will suffer with an ulcer in their lifetimes.

Fecal Occult Blood Test

This test examines the patient's stool for the presence of hidden (or occult) blood.

Procedure

A small sample of stool is obtained by the patient either at home or in the doctor's office for analysis in the laboratory.

Results

If the test indicates that there is blood present in the stool, it does not necessarily indicate cancer. A number of non-cancerous bleeding conditions, such as hemorrhoids or ulcers, may exist. This is a standard preventive or screening test often requested by doctors in the course of periodic check-ups and should not be regarded with concern.

Upper GI Series or Barium Swallow

Barium is an important element in x-ray procedures. It coats the interior of the digestive system and shows up well on x-ray film. In particular, tumors and ulcers become more apparent on x-rays using barium.

Procedure

The patient first drinks about 4 ounces of the chalky barium liquid, which is often flavored to make it more palatable. The barium coats the esophagus, stomach and small intestine. X-rays are taken as it does so and after it has had time to settle. These can be taken both sitting up and lying down. It spreads into the stomach for x-ray in about half an hour, but can take 4 hours to spread to the small intestine. The barium may cause constipation. Although the "barium cocktail" is distasteful to most patients, it is a safe and important diagnostic tool.

Results

Tumors and ulcers should stand out in the esophagus and stomach due to the outlining effect of the barium. If tumors are detected in a barium swallow procedure, a biopsy is usually required for further analysis. The extent of damage from reflux, the bubbling of stomach juices up into the esophagus, can be seen as well.

Esophageal cancer may present difficulty in swallowing. Tumorous obstructions can completely prohibit food from getting to the stomach. This cancer is more common in those over 50.

Esophagogastroduodenoscopy (EGD) or Gastroscopy or Upper GI Endoscopy

This endoscopy is often ordered when ulcers, severe heartburn, or other upper GI (gastrointestinal) disorders are present or suspected. Symptoms of these may include vomiting, especially with blood, and upper abdominal pain, or pain associated with eating and swallowing.

Procedure

The patient must usually fast for several hours beforehand to empty the stomach of all contents. The throat is anesthetized with a spray, and a sedative is given so the patient relaxes. The flexible endoscope is inserted through the mouth, down the esophagus and into the stomach and duodenum (first part of the small intestine). The interior of these organs can be examined and tests can be performed using the endoscope (see endoscopy in Medical Terms). This procedure will require 20 to 30 minutes to perform.

The duodenum refers to the first 10 inches or so of the small intestine. The pyloric sphincter, a muscle ring, connects the stomach to the duodenum and allows food to pass through at regular intervals. Ducts from the pancreas, liver and gallbladder feed bile and enzymes into the duodenum to digest food.

Results

Ulcers are the most common problem discovered during this test. They can be seen through the endoscope. Inflammation or cancers of the stomach and of the esophagus can be seen, and biopsied. This is an excellent method of finding the cause of bleeding in this part of the body. The endoscope may irritate the throat lining and leave the patient with a mild sore throat for a day or so. Because patients may require a sedative before this test, check before arriving to see if you need someone to give you a ride home.

Gastric Analysis

This test measures the amount and composition of juices in the stomach. The amount and quality of acid can help find the cause of ulcer disease or assess treatment.

Procedure

The test begins with the patient fasting up to eight hours before the test, to ensure that the stomach will be completely empty. A narrow, flexible tube is inserted through the nose and down into the stomach. Every fifteen minutes for one hour, the doctor or technician withdraws a sample of stomach juice from the tube. Then the patient is injected with a chemical that will cause the stomach to produce acid. Generally, four more samples are collected every fifteen minutes.

more tests

Results

The samples are analyzed and compared for their acid content. If the injected chemical has no effect on acid production in the stomach, this may indicate gastritis, gastric ulcer, or cancer. Increased acid in the stomach is associated with ulcers, tumors, and endocrine disease.

> Over 60 million Americans experience acid indigestion (also called Gastroesophageal Reflux Disease or GERD) at least once a month.
>
> Stomach cancer can be misdiagnosed as indigestion, and is more prevalent in those over 50. Some signs of stomach cancer: persistent feeling of fullness, pain before or after meals, change in digestion habits.
>
> Approximately 24,000 Americans are diagnosed with cancer of the stomach each year.

Helicobacter Pylori Tests

This microbe, which is recognized as contributing to gastric diseases such as duodenal ulcers, gastritis, and gastric carcinoma, can be detected by several methods, depending upon diagnostic needs.

Procedures

The helicobacter pylori bacteria is found in the mucus layer that lines the stomach and can be identified by a cultured specimen, a gastric mucosal biopsy, a blood test, or a breath test.

A biopsy or mucus specimen for culturing may be obtained by an esophagogastroduodenoscopy (EGD), as described above. The specimen should be transported to the lab within thirty minutes of collection. Analysis of blood drawn from a vein, however, is an equally accurate and simpler procedure. The breath test requires the patient to swallow a dose of radioactive C or nonradioactive C urea.

Results

A biopsy or culture will be tested for heliobacter pylori or for antibodies. Similarly, blood can be analyzed for the presence of these antibodies. The breath test is based on the ability of helicobacter pylori to break down urea into carbon dioxide and ammonia. The CO_2 concentration will reveal the presence of the microbe.

For Further Information:

National Digestive Diseases
Information Clearinghouse
2 Information Way
Bethesda, MD 20892-3570
www.niddk.nih.gov/health/digest/
pubs/diagtest/

Crohn' s & Colitis Foundation of
America, Inc.
386 Park Avenue South, 17th Floor
New York, NY 10016-8804
1-800-932-2423

American Gastrointestinal
Association
www.gastro.org

International Foundation for
Functional Gastrointestinal
Disorders (IFFGD)
P.O. Box 117864
Milwaukee, WI 53217
1-888-964-2001

The American College of
Gastroenterology (ACG)
1-800-978-7666
www.acg.gi.org/patientinfo/

Society of American Gastrointestinal
Endoscopic Surgeons (SAGES)
www.medscape.com/SAGES/
Patientinformation/pi.09.html

LOWER GI

The colon is a segmented tube approximately four and a half feet long that forms the major portion of the large intestine. It has four sections: ascending, transverse, descending, and sigmoid colon. Rhythmic contractions of the muscles along the colon push the intestinal contents through the colon to the rectum. Food has been completely digested before it enters the colon, where the primary function is to absorb water before waste leaves the body. Disorders of the colon and lower gastrointestinal system include diverticular disease, ulcerative colitis, and tumors. Diverticulosis, the formation of small sacs in the intestine which protrude from its walls, is present in half of the US population by the age of 80. This condition is permanent, and when these small sacs become inflamed (diverticulitis) the patient requires antibiotic treatment. Ulcerative colitis is an inflammation of the lining of the colon, causing bloody stool. (There are several causes of inflammation. Ulcerative colitis is only one cause.) It can lead to an increased risk of cancer, but can be treated with steroid-type drugs. The doctors who specialize in the health of the lower gastrointestinal tract are called gastroenterologists.

Colorectal cancer is one of the most common cancers. After lung cancer, it is the leading cause of cancer deaths. Incidence increases with age, beginning at about age 40. It is a common misconception that colon cancer is a disease that primarily strikes men. An equal number of men and women die from colon cancer each year. Approximately 130,000 Americans were diagnosed with the disease in 1998, half of them women. **More than 55,000 people were diagnosed too late for effective treatment and died.** Unfortunately only 20% of American adults are regularly tested for colorectal cancer.

A BITE'S PROGRESS: PART TWO

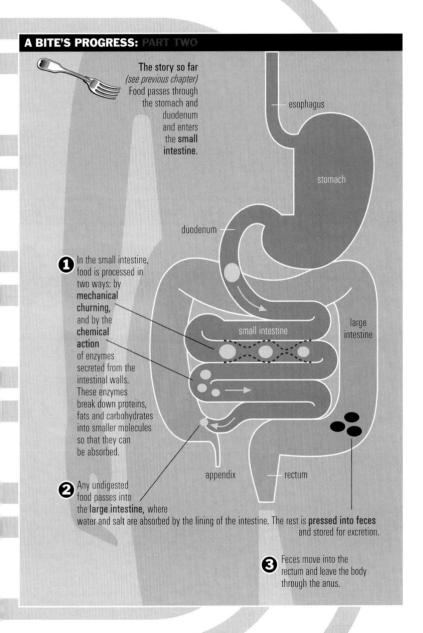

The story so far
(see previous chapter)
Food passes through the stomach and duodenum and enters the **small intestine**.

esophagus

stomach

duodenum

1 In the small intestine, food is processed in two ways: by **mechanical churning**, and by the **chemical action** of enzymes secreted from the intestinal walls. These enzymes break down proteins, fats and carbohydrates into smaller molecules so that they can be absorbed.

small intestine

large intestine

appendix

rectum

2 Any undigested food passes into the **large intestine**, where water and salt are absorbed by the lining of the intestine. The rest is **pressed into feces** and stored for excretion.

3 Feces move into the rectum and leave the body through the anus.

THE TESTS

Routine Stool Lab Tests (Occult Blood, Stool and Rectal Cultures)

Along with blood and urine, the contents of stool can provide clues to a variety of diagnoses. Like blood and urine, it is readily available and can be subjected to a battery of tests. This is one of the most common and most important tests of the lower gastrointestinal tract.

> Stool is formed through the interworkings of the intestines and the liver. Normal stool is made up of water, minerals, bile, food and bacteria.

Procedure

A stool sample provided by the patient is studied for overall appearance and then evaluated for fat content, in order to diagnose potential problems in the intestinal tract. Cultures can be conducted on stool samples to detect certain harmful bacteria, which can then be treated. Stool is also examined for parasites and blood. The presence of blood may be the first sign of a tumor, and is therefore an important diagnostic indicator. The patient should avoid red meat for two days prior to this test to avoid false positive results. Bleeding may also be caused by ASA or Motrin or other non-steroidal anti-inflammatory medications.

Results

Abnormalities in the consistency, content, odor and color of stool may reflect disease anywhere along the path food travels from top to bottom. Stool naturally contains a lot of bacteria. Some, however, are indications of abnormalities or poisons in the intestine, and these can be identified in the test. Blood in the stool, usually not evident to the naked eye, is often an indication of cancer, colitis, ulcer formation, hemorrhoids or inflammation. Stool is also examined for parasites or eggs. If blood is in the stool, this test leads to others, such as Sigmoidoscopy, Barium enema or Colonoscopy.

Proctosigmoidoscopy or Sigmoidoscopy

The purpose of this test is to see the lining of the sigmoid colon. The last 10 inches of the gastrointestinal tract are often those most plagued by disease. Frequent problems include bleeding, hemorrhoids and pain. This endoscopy examines only the lowest part of the intestinal tract. For patients over the age of 50, this test is often a preventive screening test for cancer.

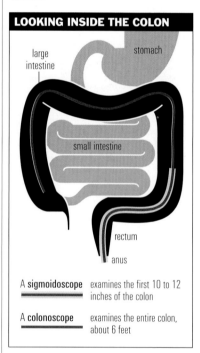

LOOKING INSIDE THE COLON

large intestine • stomach • small intestine • rectum • anus

A **sigmoidoscope** examines the first 10 to 12 inches of the colon

A **colonoscope** examines the entire colon, about 6 feet

Procedure

The patient is given oral laxatives or an enema just before the test to clear the colon. The patient then lies on an examination table, knees up to chest, as the doctor inserts the lubricated proctosigmoidoscope (a short, rigid tube) or sigmoidoscope (a 10" to 12" tube – sometimes rigid and sometimes flexible – about the size of an index finger) into the rectum. These devices differ from the colonoscope, which is a 42" to 72" flexible tube containing fiber optics. Material may be taken for biopsy as well.

Results

The doctor can see directly what may be causing the problems the patient is having. The possible diagnoses include polyps, colitis and cancer. Biopsy material can be investigated by a lab, and some growths can be removed. If something suspect is discovered, a Colonoscopy may be ordered.

THE TOP 3 REASONS TO HAVE A SIGMOIDOSCOPY

- It has been shown to locate 80% of all polyps in the colon.

- The test is associated with a 59% to 80% reduction in risk of death from cancer in the part of the colon examined.

- Periodic tests reduce anxiety about normal gastric distress.

Colonoscopy

In this test, the endoscope enters the colon through the rectum and moves up through it, examining for cancer, colitis, and polyps. The colonoscope which is used during the test is a flexible tube about as thick as an index finger which is 42" to 72" long. It contains fiber optics which light the interior of the colon for better visibility and can allow the technician to obtain computer visualizations of the colon.

Procedure

The patient takes a heavy laxative the night before the test, and cannot eat much of the day before to clear the colon completely. Sometimes additional enemas are needed. The patient lies on her left side on an examination table with knees drawn up. The doctor then lubricates and

inserts the colonoscope into the rectum. This is uncomfortable but not usually painful. Air is sometimes passed through the scope to inflate the bowel, allowing the scope to penetrate further. This causes a cramping feeling of fullness in the patient. The images transmitted from the end of the scope appear on a screen, which the doctor studies as the scope is removed. A sedative is often given to relax the patient both physically and mentally before the test. The patient may need to have a friend drive home after the test.

Results

The doctor can see any abnormalities inside the colon during this test. These include tumors, polyps, colitis and diverticular disease. Fluid samples or biopsy material gathered by the colonoscope may be analyzed for similar conditions.

Barium Enema or Air Contrast Enema

This type of x-ray is used to obtain images of the colon indirectly with x-ray films. Barium, which absorbs x-rays, lines the colon and x-rays are taken.

Each year, about 131,000 people are diagnosed with colon cancer. The cancer begins with polyps, benign, small growths on the inside of the colon. 90% of colon cancer can be cured if these polyps are removed before the cancer spreads to the lymph nodes, so early detection is key.

Procedure

The patient's colon is first cleared out, either with a laxative or by fasting, or, if needed, enemas. After a plain x-ray of the colon is taken first, the barium enema is inserted into the patient's rectum. A balloon on the enema inflates to hold it inside the

more tests ▶

rectum, and barium begins to flow into the colon. As it is distributed through the colon, additional x-ray pictures are taken. Sometimes, air is introduced through the enema as well, causing the barium to coat the colon thinly for clearer pictures. This is called an air contrast enema. The presence of barium or air produces a feeling of fullness and makes the patient feel the need to defecate immediately. It is not unusual for patients to expel some of the liquid. The patient should not feel embarrassed if this occurs. Barium will color the patient's stool light for several days, as it is expelled. The barium is safe and is not absorbed in the body.

Results

The barium makes polyps, tumors, and diverticular disease much more visible than the normal x-ray would. These problems can then be identified and treated.

Diet, body weight and physical activity all contribute to a healthy colon. A diet high in vegetables, fruits and grains, and low in animal fat will help reduce the risk. Calcium may also have a risk-reducing effect.

CT Colonoscopy

In 1996, researchers at the Bowman Gray School of Medicine in Winston-Salem, N.C. developed a new x-ray scanning procedure that is less expensive, more comfortable, and less time-consuming than barium enemas or colonoscopy. Clinical trials are under way to determine whether this technique is effective. Until these studies are completed, this procedure should not be considered a standard of care.

Procedure

After the patient has had cleansing enemas or has fasted, air is inserted into the colon. A helical CT scanner passing painlessly over the patient requires less than two minutes to gather two-dimensional images that can be reconstructed to show doctors and technicians views of the colon that are sliced vertically, horizontally, and in cross-section.

Results

The images from the CT scan reveal all polyps that are larger than one centimeter in size and most other smaller polyps. Polyps larger than one centimeter have a higher likelihood of becoming cancerous. A three-dimensional version of this same technology, known as a virtual colonoscopy, is under development. This would provide views as though a camera were travelling through the colon.

Laparoscopy

This type of endoscopy is used to examine unexplained abdominal pain. The procedure allows the doctor to see the outer surface of all the abdominal organs.

Procedure

The lower abdomen is cleaned and sterilized, and general anesthesia is administered. A small incision is made in the skin and the laparoscope slipped inside. The scope is then used to observe and test the internal organs as during any endoscopy. The scope will be used to fill the abdominal cavity with air, making viewing easier.

Results

From this perspective, doctors can detect cancers and liver disease. It lets them have direct observation of these organs. Any fluid collected or biopsy material can also be analyzed.

Carcinoembryonic Antigen Blood Test (CEA)

Seventy percent of patients with

colon cancer have an elevated level of this antigen in their blood.

Procedure

Blood is drawn from a vein and sent to a lab for analysis.

Results

Although this is helpful in following known cases of colon cancer, it is not a good screening test. The antigen is also elevated in cases of cancers elsewhere in the body and in the blood of smokers. It is often used to monitor therapy and detect a recurrence of cancer as well.

Rectal Digital Examination

This test is a quick and simple way to screen for both colon cancer and polyps (which can turn into colon cancer). It is most often performed as part of a routine pelvic exam because it also checks for tumors on the wall between the colon and the vagina.

Procedure

The doctor wears sterile latex gloves, and, using one finger, he probes and touches the anal area and the entrance to the rectum.

Results

The doctor may also note the presence of hemorrhoidal tissues or scarring in the rectal area. In addition, any polyps or growths detected in the rectum might require removal or biopsy for further diagnosis.

For Further Information

National Cancer Information Service
9000 Rockville Pike
Bethesda, MD 20892
301-496-4000

Agency for Health Care Policy and Research Publications Clearinghouse
P.O. Box 8547
Silver Spring, MD 20907
1-800-358-9295
www.ahcpr.gov/

National Digestive Diseases Information Clearinghouse
2 Information Way
Bethesda, MD 20892-3570
www.niddk.nih.gov/health/digest/pubs/diagtest/

American Gastrointestinal Association
www.gastro.org/

The American College of Gastroenterology (ACG)
1-800-978-7666
www.acg.gi.org/patientinfo/

Society of American Gastrointestinal Endoscopic Surgeons (SAGES)
www.medscape.com/SAGES/Patientinformation/pi.09.html

REPRODUCTIVE SYSTEM

The female reproductive system is literally the cradle of human life.

Except for the vulva or outside, it lies entirely within the pelvic cavity, well protected from many physical dangers. The ovaries produce and release eggs on a monthly cycle. The eggs travel through the fallopian tubes into the uterus or womb, where implantation occurs. The entrance to the uterus is called the cervix; it leads into the vagina, which in turn leads out of the body through the vulva.

The ovaries also secrete hormones, estrogen and progesterone, which regulate the female reproductive cycle. Typically a woman ovulates, or releases one egg every 28 days. If unfertilized, it is passed out of the body along with the lining of the uterus, through the process of menstruation. If fertilized, the egg attaches itself to the uterine wall and the woman is pregnant. Pregnancy and childbirth have a powerful impact on the female reproductive system, including

THE TOP 5 QUESTIONS TO ASK YOUR DOCTOR ABOUT REPRODUCTIVE TESTS

? If I have a pain or discomfort that I think originates in my reproductive organs, what should I do right away?

? What is the best test to diagnose my particular symptons?

? If there is a possibility that I am pregnant, are there particular tests that should be avoided?

? What are the recent variations on the Pap Test that may affect my results?

? How can I deal with the embarrassment or psychological discomfort about gynecological tests?

physical and hormonal changes. Menstruation begins at puberty and ends with menopause, signaling the completion of the reproductive years. The doctor who treats female reproductive organs is an obstetrician/gynecologist. There are specialists within obstetrics and gynecology, such as obstetricians, who deal with pregnancy, and gynecological oncologists, who deal with cancer of the female reproductive system.

Women should have an annual gynecological exam, including a Pap test. The doctor should ask questions about sexual history, menstrual regularity, use of birth control, and pregnancy. In addition to a physical examination including the patient's breasts, the clinician should instruct her on how to conduct a breast self-exam (see diagram on page 56). Gynecological offices may perform mammograms, or may refer the patient to another facility (hospital, lab, or clinic) where mammograms are performed. In addition to the annual check-up, an obstetrician/gynecologist should be consulted if a woman is planning on getting pregnant, or if she suspects that she has contracted a sexually transmitted disease (STD).

Tests of the reproductive organs are necessary for routine preventive health, as well as for detection of problems associated with pregnancy or menopause. It is normal for women to experience gynecological problems at some point in their lives, but these problems are usually not life-threatening. The greatest health risks for the reproductive organs are sexually transmitted diseases (STDs) and cancer. According to the Centers for Disease Control and Prevention, 15 million Americans become infected with an STD each year. Sexually active teenagers are particularly at risk. One in ten adolescent girls tested for chlamydia is infected.

WHY IS IT CALLED A "PAP" TEST

The test is named after George Papanicolaou, who developed it in 1928.

Since the introduction of the Pap test, deaths from cervical cancer have dropped 70%, but it is still one of the leading causes of cancer deaths for women. Of the 5,000 women who die from cervical cancer each year, 50% have not had a Pap test done in five or more years.

Tragically, 50% of women over age 65 do not have regular Pap smears or mammograms.

THE TESTS

GENITAL ORGANS

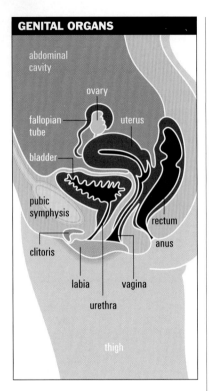

- abdominal cavity
- ovary
- fallopian tube
- uterus
- bladder
- pubic symphysis
- rectum
- anus
- clitoris
- labia
- vagina
- urethra
- thigh

Pelvic Examination

An examination of a woman's external and internal reproductive organs is performed as a preventive part of a complete physical examination or in response to abdominal pain, vaginal bleeding, urinary incontinence or infertility. It is an important test for identifying prolapsed uterus, ovarian cysts, and other problems. This examination may be conducted by the primary care physician or an obstetrician/gynecologist.

Procedure

The woman is asked to lie on her back with her knees bent or to be seated in a gynecological examination chair. The doctor will first inspect the external genitals for signs of ulceration, swelling, sores, or other abnormalities. Then, a speculum, a device used to hold open the vaginal walls, is inserted to allow a clear view of the vagina and the cervix, the neck of the uterus. The speculum may be made of plastic or metal. It may be

shaped like a duck's bill with wide curved edges, or like a shoehorn bent at both ends. With the speculum in place, the doctor will make a visual determination of the health of the tissues and the condition of these areas. Wearing a plastic or latex glove, the doctor will insert two fingers into the vagina to feel the size and position of the uterus and ovaries and to detect any abnormal pelvic swelling or growth.

Results

This simple physical examination provides the doctor with an overview of the health of a woman's reproductive system, and is the basis for consideration of further testing or analysis.

"PAP TALK"

Your doctor may use some of these abbreviations in explaining the results of your test:

- ASCUS — Atypical Squamous Cells of Undetermined Significance: Some slight abnormalities that may be caused by HPV wart virus and will require further observation.
- AGUS — Atypical Glandular Cells of Undetermined Significance: Slight abnormalities which may indicate infection or inflamation of glands.
- LSIL — Low-grade Squamous Intraepithelial Lesion—A common condition which sometimes suggests the presence of the Human Papilloma Virus (HPV) wart virus.

Pap Test or Pap Smear

This test for cervical cancer is part of every gynecological annual exam. It can detect cervical cancer earlier than any other method, and is most often performed on healthy women as a routine preventive procedure.

Procedure

The patient reclines on the examination table, with her feet in the stirrups or in a gynecological examina-

